# *DMD Life*

## art and me

*by*

### Ian A. Griffiths

Grosvenor House
Publishing Limited

This book is published by
Grosvenor House Publishing Ltd
28-30 High Street, Guildford, Surrey, GU1 3HY.
www.grosvenorhousepublishing.co.uk

A CIP record for this book
is available from the British Library

ISBN 978-1-907652-33-2

This book is dedicated to my dear friend and brother in Duchenne Sam Morgan. He was sadly and cruelly taken in September 2010 by the deadly claw of this muscle disease. Your kind, loving and brave soul will be fondly remembered ever more. The painting on the back cover was painted especially for him, may he now walk above the clouds. My thoughts go out especially to Sam's parents Debbie and Colin.

# *Foreword*

I'm Ian Griffiths from South Wales. This book is a story of my life so far up to the age of twenty five years. I live with and suffer from the ill effects of DMD which stands for Duchenne Muscular Dystrophy. It is a severe muscle wasting disease and a life limiting terminal illness. It won't kill you in six months in the traditional sense of 'terminal', but it's far crueller than that, it steals every muscle in your body first and then kills you, anywhere up to the age of thirty. There have been cases of men living past that into their forties and fifties but only with drastic interventions such as ventilators and tracheotomies, more on this can be found by reading on.

I hope to cover a few things in this book, from a history of my childhood years to a more detailed history from sixteen years onwards and finally onto my current problems and triumphs. At times things I write may make you smile or may make you pause and think about the seriousness of life with this devastating disease. I really hope there will be a cure but currently for us supposedly 'older' guys with DMD (over twenty one), there seems very little hope. If I don't see a cure in my lifetime, I hope my campaigning helps in some way bring it about for future generations, so another child won't have to see their body wither and die before their time

# Table of Contents

# TABLE OF CONTENTS

# A History of my Childhood Years – Diagnosis

It all started on a summers' afternoon, I was born on the fourteenth of July 1984 at around two fifteen in the afternoon in East Glamorgan hospital, South Wales. This happened to be Bastille Day a French holiday; it must have been why I liked the language later on in school. I appeared to be a 'normal' healthy child who weighed in at seven pounds twelve ounces. My mother often says I was born needing a shave and a haircut!

My parents and sisters took me home, which at the time was in Treforest to a small terraced house. I don't remember much of my time in Treforest as we moved when I was only one year old. My mother is Susan known to most as Sue a short dark haired bespectacled lady, she originally came from Abercynon and worked as a bank clerk, she's currently my main carer. My father is Tony he's from Penrhiwceiber, a tall imposing brown haired man. At the time he worked in UWIST whilst studying toward his PhD, and he's now a Professor at Cardiff University. He is a chartered engineer but his current field is Mechanical Engineering, most notably waste management. My eldest sister is Emma; she was six years old in 1984 and is now a tall, dark haired lady with two children. My middle sister is Sian; she was nearly two years old in 1984 and is now of average height with blonde hair. Emma currently works as a school teacher in a special school. Sian currently works as a teaching assistant in a special school.

After a year we moved back to my mothers' old house in Abercynon, a little while after her parents had passed away. She and my father bought the house from her sister Cheryl and her husband Martin. Their parents left the house between the two of them and because Cheryl had her own house my parents were able to buy her out. It is a normal sized terraced house on a very pleasant street, not far from a small park, where I used to hang out. Abercynon is a small village not far from Pontypridd in the Cynon valley. It is divided in two by the river Cynon with a bridge crossing it; we call the part across the river the 'other side'. Over the other side is the main shopping area with a baker, chip shop, a few pubs, a post office and the railway station. On the near side of Abercynon there are a lot of houses and two schools; a Welsh speaking and an English speaking school. There's a small shop and a busy road as you enter Abercynon. We used to have a butcher but the recent recession signalled the final whistle on that. Also we are surrounded by the greenery and rolling hills of the South Wales valleys. To get your bearings, Brecon is a few miles to the North and Cardiff is a further few miles to the South.

When I was about 18 months old my mother noticed I wasn't moving around like I should have been, my sisters could run rings around me. I was often bumping into things and holding on to furniture whilst walking.

My mother was obviously concerned, so she contacted the health visitor and our family doctor. They were unconcerned at first and didn't know why I was having trouble walking. My mother then had to persuade them to let me be seen by a paediatrician, they had put my problems down to over worrying on my mothers' part, but after a few weeks they finally relented. I was seen at Aberdare hospital by the paediatrician who was then in charge.

During the consultation they took a blood sample from me and soon the paediatrician saw the results. These showed extremely high Creatine Kinase levels and he thought I had something called Muscular Dystrophy, but he wasn't really confident of a diagnosis. Creatine Kinase is an enzyme, which when released in elevated levels could indicate amongst other things muscle disease. A few weeks later my parents were told to take me for a muscle biopsy at the University hospital of Wales, Cardiff.

The biopsy was scheduled soon after, however it was in the days before keyhole surgery, so they had to cut into my thigh and remove a muscle sample. My parents must have been very worried and alarmed by this. They don't say much about that time, but would answer any questions I had. I find it difficult to talk about that time myself, as it must have been a difficult emotional period for my family.

The night after the biopsy whilst soundly asleep in my bed the stitches burst from the wound and blood must have poured absolutely everywhere! I can only imagine the noise I must have made screaming, all I can vaguely remember is the agony I felt all night long. It turned out that the biopsy site had become infected and after a course of antibiotics I soon healed as best I could but the damage was done. I'm now left with a scar on my right thigh over an inch long, it doesn't look so bad these days but it was another painful reminder of things to come.

After that seriously painful night a few more weeks passed until the day we received a letter. It told us to go back to the hospital in Aberdare. My parents and I, along with my sisters made our way to Aberdare hospital. I can only assume they were apprehensive on the one hand and relieved on the other hand to at last find out why I was having so much trouble moving and walking.

Once in Aberdare we were kept waiting for quite some time, my parents were offered tea, a very British way of dealing with bad news. Eventually we were ushered into the paediatrician's room; according to my mother his name was Dr. Maguire, a tall bespectacled man who appeared dapper. My parents were offered a seat whilst my sisters and I played with the toys oblivious to the gravity of the situation. It was explained to my parents that my biopsy result came back positive for a disease called Duchenne Muscular Dystrophy (often abbreviated DMD). He didn't really explain to my parents what it was, only to tell them it was a muscle wasting condition. So in great shock and despair my parents took us home, still none the wiser about this DMD condition that their son was unaware of; as he happily played with his toys.

My parents' were not content just knowing the name of my condition, so they asked Dr. Maguire if he could recommend any expert on muscle disease. After awhile we were sent to see a Professor (at that time he was a doctor) Sibert, he knew a lot more about Duchenne's than the local paediatrician did. An appointment was made shortly after. We all had to proceed to the medical genetics department in the University hospital of Wales, Cardiff. I can only remember it was a modern department with plenty of toys a toddler would be happy with. It had the usual white walls and that pungent disinfectant odour you can smell for days. We were shown into a room and there sat a tall portly man with a beard wearing a dark suit. He introduced himself as Dr. Sibert to my parents; he then set about telling them what Duchenne Muscular Dystrophy was.

Duchenne Muscular Dystrophy is a rare (approx. 1 in 3500 births in the UK) severe terminal muscle wasting genetic disease that gradually kills all the body's muscle cells. Firstly it attacks the skeletal muscles, especially the legs, hips, arms and spine. It quickly moves on to abdominal muscles, meaning boys are usually in a wheelchair between the ages of seven to ten. Finally it attacks the heart and respiratory muscles. Eventually leading to an early death due to cardiac or respiratory arrest, at the time in 1986 the average life expectancy was only twelve years! There is no cure. (These days it's nearer twenty, because of serious medical interventions. However many children are still dying and a cure is still elusive.)

My parents' world must have absolutely crashed around them and it was definitely the lowest time of their lives. After hearing the average life expectancy of twelve years they were in immense shock. How could their son, who was happily playing with plastic cars, possibly die at such a young age? My mother has told me recently that at that very moment, she was still confused and had almost no understanding of this rare condition. She was astounded to find no help anywhere; there wasn't even a proper counsellor.

In case you're wondering what causes Duchenne Muscular dystrophy, I will explain it in terms of how it affects me. There is a protein called Dystrophin located in everyone's DNA, that is missing or damaged in an affected male, it affects mainly males because it's an X linked recessive error; males only have one X chromosome. This causes the muscle fibre membranes (Dystrophin acts as a shock absorber) to get over-stressed and die off, releasing Creatine Kinase into the bloodstream. Eventually the dead cells get turned into connective tissue and adipose (fatty compounds). At a genetic level, I have something called Exon fifty missing, which is known as a deletion. Exons' are like letters or words in a genetic "sentence". For instance say the normal "sentence" for Dystrophin is;

THE CAT AND TOM RUN FAR

In the case of my deletion the "sentence" looks like this; (imagine the letter "e" represents Exon fifty)

THC ATA NDT OMR UNF ARA

(more info here- MDEX consortium http://www.mdex. org.uk in their FAQ area) This obviously makes no sense and is thus called a 'nonsense mutation' by geneticists.

This fault in the 'reading' frame of Dystrophin causes my DMD. There are other causes of DMD but my knowledge of those is not comprehensive enough. DMD varies in severity and a much less severe type is called Becker's Muscular Dystrophy.

After a few quiet moments we all left the warm office, I was upset to leave the toys. I never for once thought anything was wrong, oblivious to this monster on my back which was going to rob me of everything. Driving back home my parents must have had their dreams smashed, my father wouldn't get to see me play rugby, wouldn't see me taking part in all the normal things people take for granted. My mother wouldn't see her boy grow to be an old man and probably wouldn't see him getting married or having a child. They would see me possibly die young or live and suffer. Which would you prefer? I often wonder.

Once we got home my mother's defences broke and she cried at the devastating news. Living a life not many people would comprehend. The next day, while I was lining up toy cars on the floor, my mother looked everywhere to find some support. She couldn't find any for weeks; help seemed so elusive. Finally she found a muscle disease charity which gave her much needed information on DMD; she joined their membership scheme shortly after. She fundraised with them for a good few years. After the information sunk in, it was decided by my parents that if I only had 12 years to live. They would give me the best and fulfilled twelve years they could. So started my life with the monster, it's now DMD and me!

# *After Diagnosis*

A few months after that devastating day in 1986 I had started at a local primary school in Abercynon called Abertaf. My parents were advised by Dr. Maguire to send me to a 'special' school, but my father flatly refused that idea. I did not appear to have any developmental problems. Also (I'm grateful to say) he wanted me to learn geography, history, maths and all the other subjects so called 'normal' children take. Not learn to "tie my laces", even though I would have been too weak to do that later in life. I was going to be 'different' enough without going to a special school. Abertaf is a local mainstream primary school, which is a good ten minutes walk from my house.

I made a lot of friends and my best friend at the time was a lovely girl called Elizabeth, who seemed so much taller than me; she had short hair and spectacles. I have wonderful memories of starting school remembering long hazy days, crunching through colourful autumn leaves and watching my breath freeze in the biting cold of winter. I often waved my mother goodbye each morning, unlike many of the other children I never cried when I saw her walk up the hill to go home. I was just so excited to be in school and very eager to learn all that new information.

Meanwhile unbeknownst to me, my mother had lots of trouble with some other rather ignorant parents. They could see I had major trouble moving and they could also see me interacting with their children. On many occasions they have asked "Is he contagious? Will my kid get that?" My mother always answered calmly (I don't know how, in the face of such indignance) that I have a genetic disease that is most certainly not contagious.

It was so hard for her constantly allaying other peoples' fears and misgivings, when what she really needed at that time was support and understanding. I am really angry when I think back, at what my mother and family had to endure. Other terminal illnesses are met with some sort of instant empathy, with tears and hugs thrown in too. My illness is met with suspicion and a total lack of knowledge or worse still they think you're "putting it on". It's important for people not to judge when or if they know a child has a DMD, the best thing you can do in my opinion is to say you're sorry to hear of the devasting news. Also ask is there anything you can do to help. Please try not to ask questions that you wouldn't ask of any other terminally or seriously ill patient.

By the time I was four to five years old a lot of things were starting to happen at home and at school. I was getting noticeably slower and weaker in school; the headmaster was quite helpful and got the LEA (Local Educational Authority) to install ramps and an improved toilet area for when I would need a wheelchair. At home my parents' were advised to get an extension put onto our house and to install a lift. There was a grants procedure to help out with some of the costs, but my father had to pay for certain extras; plans were started shortly after.

Most parents were getting the message that I wasn't contagious, but my mother and I still got silly questions directed at us. Such as "Why is he in a buggy?" and "He should be walking, not pushed in the shopping trolley!" even though my muscles were dying in front of these people. We developed a thick skin and I've been positive about most of my disease ever since then. Although I can't be one hundred percent positive all the time, it's not humanly possible!

At around six years old I would get extremely tired by the end of the day; my mother had to get me taxis to and from school. I got an assistant at school, to supervise me and to help with my classroom activities. Every six months I was going to the muscle clinic led by doctor Sibert to get progress updates, they would check how far I could walk before getting tired. My lung capacity was checked with a peak flow meter, you basically blow into a device that has an arrow moved by the air you expel. The end you blow into looks and feels like the inside cardboard roll of a toilet paper roll. As you can imagine this is not the most appealing thing for a child to want to go near!

Often the doctor's and physiotherapists would stretch my legs, feet and arms. I can only ever remember the pain, it would make me cry out and hot tears would run down my cheeks. I understood that I needed to endure this because my legs were very weak, but I still hated it. It was extremely frightening and I often went very quiet during the car journey home. My legs were really tight and sensitive to pressure so my mother was told to stretch me everyday. I had to endure this pain everyday, some days I would just get so fed up and angry of Duchenne's that I would argue and bargain just not to do them. Mostly though I just got on with it, the pain wasn't too unbearable after a few weeks, it was my new routine. I had to have stretches done in school by my assistant; there was no escape from this disease.

My father would take my sisters and I horse riding every Saturday. We went to a local country park which had a stable run by a charity called "Riding for the Disabled", I loved riding a small horse called Gladys she was very gentle and always behaved. There have been times when I was thrown off another horse but this was rare and thankfully I never broke any bones. I must have just bounced off the ground! I could only ride until I was around twelve years old because of a complete lack of balance caused by my DMD.

A funny moment my family and I often discuss was during one cold winter's day. I was out riding; my father and cousin Sarah were walking beside me. After a gentle ride past some snow banks the horse suddenly got startled and threw me off! I landed in some soft snow in a daze. My cousin was standing there laughing as my father chased after the bolting horse, I can remember his hat falling off and flapping behind him in a comical manner. He finally found the horse in a field. It was trying to catch up to some other galloping horses! If only we had a camera, there was no YouTube then unfortunately.

Every Sunday until I was about sixteen years old my parents took me swimming at a local pool. My dad setup a swimming charity called 'Cynon Valley Starfish' local children with disabilities attended. I had many people help me while I was swimming, I needed supervision just incase I couldn't right myself. A friend of the family called Matthew (a tall dark haired slightly balding man who has a very quick wit) used to watch over me. He would throw me across the pool, which always made me laugh. I used to mess about a lot when Matt was supervising; he was and still is funny. However if my father was supervising I'd have to do some swimming to get my exercise in. We'd do several lengths of the pool; I could do it easily at a young age.

In my later swimming years my father would drag me around the pool with his feet under my arms so I could join in with the lengths. It was a happy time that all the family joined in with, including my mother who would watch us through a large window sitting in a small cafeteria. We could earn swimming badges ranging from red to blue badges, I think blue badges were the hardest of all to get. You needed to be able to take off wet clothes whilst swimming and swim various distances in a set time to get a blue badge. I can only remember one boy who was blind ever earning that accolade. I managed to get two badges a red and yellow one, I was always happy with my two little square badges. I could never get those last two badges, it was yet another small thing that DMD robbed me of, I would never have the strength to complete the tests involved. A great plus side however was that my legs got much needed exercise without fighting against gravity.

I was always sleepy after my swims probably due to a freezing cold pool. I feel the cold very badly these days, I suspect the reason behind this is the fact I can't move anymore (I'm often found swathed in fleece covers and wraps; our heating is on throughout the year too!). We always had chocolate or crisps in the cafeteria afterwards to warm up a bit; my mother would give me a bite of her *Ruffle* chocolate bar. We got home by five p.m. and my father would watch *Wildlife on one*. This was so boring to me that I wasn't long drifting off to sleep in my comfortable bed. A time when I could truly escape, dreaming of winning sports contests and climbing mountains, but sadly I had to wake up weak again. That is a measure of the truly heartbreaking nature of Duchenne's muscular dystrophy. I always try to fixate on the things I can do and that makes it a tiny bit easier to get through the depressing times.

# Age Seven to Eight

As I approached my seventh birthday on this Earth my deterioration was running away at a great pace. Walking was becoming very difficult. I can remember walking with hands held above my head supported by my school assistant. This was in order to keep my balance; it was an extremely slow way of walking. If I fell as I often did, there was no way of me getting up, I'd need help. I was very frustrated and upset by this tiring, ungainly way of moving. I remember one time being pushed over by a young girl and falling flat on my face unfortunately I bit into my tongue producing a huge gash. It was extremely hard to talk for a few days but luckily I healed up, it was yet more reminders of my Duchenne's induced weakness.

At home things were dramatically changing around me. Doors were widened; the extension had been completed and we now had a larger bathroom and a larger back bedroom. My first lift was being built out of tubular steel; I often looked up the lift shaft, it went right to the attic ceiling. The lift was a large metal box, with a sliding metal door and was powered by a chain driven motor. It took about sixty seconds to get from the ground floor to the first floor. It was quite noisy but got the job done.

There was a huge fuss made by the council, originally they wanted us to have the lift installed in our living room! That would have been highly inappropriate and would have blocked the light entering through our front window. It would be difficult welcoming people into your main living area with a hulking steel box in the way. We really had to fight to get it changed. My dad had to pay to make sure the lift went in the new extended area. I really hope things have changed on the grants front, so you don't need to pay just to get around your own house.

In school I had a sloping wooden table made to help my posture and make writing easier. It was custom made by a firm in a town called Llantrisant; "*Traditional toys*" was its name. They made a lot of wooden items for children. It was beautifully assembled and made my life a lot easier. I enjoyed learning in school and this only enhanced my experiences. I would recommend them fully to someone in a similar position as I.

I remember when our class had an Egyptian day; we all dressed up in sheets, and ate dates. We tried all sorts of foods from the area and drew many wonderful drawings of pyramids and sunny blue skies. I think we also watched a video about Egypt. Other lessons I remember were notable in teaching me about geology; we got to see a rock collection, including granite, pumice and various other small semi-precious gems. Also I learned about sound, the class was shown a video of a drum which had grains of sand on it. When it was tapped, you could see the grains explode off the drum, the video explained about sound waves vibrating when the drummer tapped on it. Embarrassingly when I saw the grains leap from the drum I shouted out "Wow!" the teacher told me off with a sharp "Ian! Shhh" I was very excited, it sparked an interest in science I've had to this day.

By my eighth birthday I suffered a giant set back that made that particular year the hardest in my short life so far. It was a sunny day and I got up early as I usually did. I'd been falling a lot for a few days prior so I was taking it slowly walking around. I went down the stairs on my backside because it would hurt my legs doing it the conventional way. I walked slowly towards the kitchen and saw my breakfast waiting for me. It was probably toast, as cereal wasn't my absolute favourite food. Eating at seven or eight in the morning wasn't very appealing as it made me feel sick most days, so toast was a safer choice than anything else.

After I'd finished my breakfast I walked into the living room to watch my favourite cartoons on the television, "*teenage mutant hero turtles*" was the real "in" thing, so naturally I loved them. I had many figurines and tons of *VHS* videos stacked up around the house. A few minutes later I'd finished watching the cartoons, and for some unknown reason, I decided to walk around an armchair we had. Perhaps it was a game or a bit of exercise, I can't really remember.

As I was milling around the chair my knees suddenly buckled and I fell hard to the floor. I cried out to my mother that something was wrong. She came rushing over and tried to help me up, but it was hopeless. No matter what she tried I could not stand, I just couldn't bear any weight. My legs felt heavy and totally useless,

I could have cried my heart out as I struggled but I just forced my tears back. I remember being so terribly upset and distressed, I shouted at my mother and she shouted back. I could tell she was as upset and distressed as I was but she remained calm for my sake. Finally we had to get my oversized blue and white buggy that I'd had since I was five, my mother got me into it lifting and pulling me up as she went. At least I was a bit more comfortable for the time being as a cold numbness crept over me, invading every orifice.

DMD had cruelly and selfishly robbed me of my legs! It's a never ending progression, a constant domino effect. Its ever increasing grip over me had finally overwhelmed my legs; it's these things that really make you intensely dislike this disease. Various expletives couldn't even begin to describe how Duchenne's makes you feel, and that's no exaggeration! I could scream at this disease all day and still feel no better. This is one of the hardest times for me to go over, but it is part of my life none the less. I just wanted to shout and cry, but I figured what's the use. I was exhausted by my efforts anyway.

I just sat in my buggy for awhile, quietly contemplating what would happen next. I think I watched some television for a few more minutes. Quickly my mother had to arrange a wheelchair for me. I think I got an NHS (National Health Service) wheelchair sent over not long after. It was a huge clunky thing that weighed a ton. It was made of grey tubular steel and black leather, it had the ability to rise into a standing position but my muscles were too weak for me to use it. It looked terrible but it was my new 'legs' for the time being.

I had to have additional equipment added to my house, so I could be transferred from a wheelchair to my bed; also to get on the toilet and in my bathtub. I had two ceiling hoists installed. It would take a few years before I needed them. In the meantime my mother or father would have to lift or carry me from my wheelchair to the bed or toilet. This was very hard on us all, I'd lost my independence, and they put their backs in danger. Also I was ordered a new "mobile" hoist, one which could be wheeled around, but again that would take a few years to arrive.

While the world welcomed in the 1990's, saw the Berlin wall fall and the end of Soviet Union. I was dealing with a body blow on my own. I never knew any other lad's in my situation at that time. Apart from my family I was totally alone. For an eight year old to suddenly be walking one minute and immobile the next you would have thought I would get some professional support. There was no counselling offered, no emotional support in school, there was nothing, (this nothingness would become a recurring feature of my future healthcare). I just had to get on with it, struggling through each day. I thought there's one of two ways to go, either I get really angry and cry everyday or I think as positively as I can. I chose to think positively, see what I could do and concentrate on that. It worked for me, but I had to bottle a lot of emotions up as there was no-one to really discuss them with. I think sheer will power and a loving family got me through. I even started to like my wheels.

Soon after that terrible business I got a much cooler wheelchair which I could push around myself, but that didn't last long however. DMD was now busily attacking my arm muscles which meant I couldn't push myself any longer. I had to get an electric wheelchair, which was provided by a charity. The one fitted for me was excellent; it even had a bright red comfortable cushion. I didn't take long to adjust to it. I loved going outside in it, feeling the speed push me over the pavement and up hills. It was only five miles per hour but to me it felt like fifty! I often drove up the hill outside my house to go and see a large fish pond a neighbour had. The Koi carp would glisten in the glorious sunshine we occasionally had, it was mesmerising for an eight year old.

I can only remember one major incident whilst driving. I was on my own driving up the hill outside my house when suddenly the chair stopped. I was stuck; I checked the controls and tapped it a few times. Still no power lights were showing. The only thing that it could have been was a loose cable. I tried calling my mother but the house was too far away. I started to panic, but eventually managed to calm myself. Ten minutes later a couple of ladies appeared wearing brightly coloured clothes, they were walking up the street towards their house I can only assume.

Instinctively I called out "Excuse me! Can I have some help please?" luckily the younger of the two ladies came over and saw a wire hanging loose from my battery. She plugged it back in and my power lights flickered back into life. I breathed a huge sigh of relief and thanked the kind lady. I then went on my way slowly avoiding the bumps on the uneven pavement. I got back home a few minutes later saying very little to my mother. The joys of electric wheelchairs! This only showed me that going out unsupervised wasn't exactly a good idea, but while I could, I did venture out there.

Even more this insidious condition was stealing my muscles. It's amazing what the body can deal with, but how much more could I take. I felt my will power and determination would see me through any upcoming troubles, but the truth is no-one knows what's ahead of them.

# Meeting the Prime Minister

A fabulous distraction to losing my mobility was offered by a charity called the "*Starlight Children's Foundation*", they were setup to grant wishes to seriously and terminally ill children, to take their mind off (however briefly) their conditions and illnesses. My wish for some reason was to meet the then Prime Minister Sir John Major. I suppose I just wanted to meet the leader of the government and visit London, the capital city of Great Britain.

My parents', sisters and I all set off from Cardiff by train bound for Piccadilly station. It was a great journey; I can remember playing *Tetris* on my new *Game boy* for most of the way. I used to challenge my father to a high score contest, I always wanted to win. I'm still very competitive when it comes to gaming! A few hours later the train rolled to a stop and everyone disembarked onto a very busy platform. After we got off the train we had to get a black cab to take us to Downing Street. I drove my electric wheelchair up two small metal ramps into the cab; my father loaded our luggage and off we went to Downing Street. I was getting excited and nervous all at the same time. I was noticeably quiet while the taxi jostled through the busy London traffic; after quite some time we pulled up a few metres outside that famous street in Whitehall.

My mother and I were the only two allowed to see the Prime Minister. My father and sisters went shopping while we were in number ten. We met up with a lovely lady from the "*Starlight Foundation*" called Cheryl a tall blonde bespectacled woman who was sharply dressed in grey. Coincidentally she shared the same name as my aunty. The three of us made our way to number ten and when we arrived there was a photographer waiting. The policeman on the door helped get my wheelchair up over the step and my mother and I posed for our picture.

Once inside the very palatial building, I was ushered over to a lift. It must have been the smallest lift in the world! I don't know how my wheelchair fitted in to it. My driving skills must have advanced exponentially during that manoeuvre. Soon I was on the upper floor and my next obstacle was five small steps. About four or five burly men lifted my chair and I over the steps. Those guys would have been incredibly helpful back at home I thought. I drove through wonderfully decorated rooms and carefully avoided some large antique furniture. Next I went into the cabinet room as seen on television which was dominated by a large table and many chairs. It was so exciting for a common boy from the South Wales valleys. Next thing I knew I was being whisked into see the Prime Minister.

I went through a large shiny black door into an office type room which was ornately decorated. There sat Prime Minister John Major in front of a huge window, he was wearing a snappy black suit with a slender tie and his glasses glinted in the over head lighting. I went really shy but finally managed to say a meek "Hello". He knew my name and nearly pronounced Abercynon correctly (Aber Kun Non being the correct pronunciation) I was totally blown away by this. I never knew Prime Minister's had aides back then. It felt like some kind of magic to me and I certainly couldn't understand where he got his information from.

I brought along a present for him; it was an exquisite painting/etching of a coal mine pit head. We handed it over to him; he was very polite and graciously accepted my gift. I also got a present back; an impressive gold medallion, which came in a wonderfully green lined velvet box. It shined brightly in the sun, as I played with it in my hands. I talked a little bit about my disease, but I didn't know a great deal then. Except that it was making me weaker of course. After some more pleasantries and insightful conversation my mother and I "stood" next to Sir Major and again posed for pictures. Two photographs still hang in my blue walled bedroom they are glass fronted and surrounded by green framing.

Our visit was fast running down and it was time to leave the Prime Minister to get on with domestic affairs (no pun intended). My mother led the way back to the five steps and again the helpful men lifted my chair and I down. I drove to the smallest elevator in the world and made my way to the ground floor. I arrived with a thud and drove toward the shiny black door out into the light; I think my photograph was taken again. I'd bought a fantastic new black and white shirt for the day, so I really didn't mind being photographed at all!

Outside the gates we were met by the taxi; my sisters and father were waiting for us. Once I got up the metal ramps and into the taxi; my mother and I were given one beautifully moist baguette each. It was very welcome as we were famished after our wonderful trip to number ten Downing Street. We then set off towards our hotel which at that time was called "*The Moat House*" in Covent Garden. Awhile later we arrived outside the hotel; it was a really pleasant building with beautiful stonework. We all got out of the taxi and made our way to the foyer. My father quickly received the room key and we all boarded a big elevator. It quietly whisked us to our floor; opening with a ping we saw a plush carpeted corridor. My wheelchair battery lights were flashing; indicating to me that it was recharging time.

My father opened the door onto a medium sized room, and I slowly edged my chair into a space by a big bed. I was tired and wanted to stretch out, so my mother helped lift me onto the bed. The wheelchair was charged while I was resting. My sisters Emma and Sian showed me what they had bought whilst I was with the Prime Minister. Emma had some new jeans and Sian had some new tops. They had bought me two new games for my *Game boy*. I remember having the games "*Asteroids*" and "*Universal Soldier*". *Asteroids* was my favourite, I loved shooting at the tiny rocks whizzing around the small green LCD screen. *Universal Soldier* was a far more complicated shooting game that I gave up on after awhile.

A few hours later I was getting thirsty, so my mother rang for room service to bring up a glass of cola for me. Two or so minutes later a young impatient man came up with my cola in a tall glass with some ice bobbing around in it. He says to me "Young man, get up and take your drink! There's nothing wrong with you helping your mother out" he was quite condescending and hurtful in his tone. My mother was shocked by this and stepped in, pointing at my wheelchair; he suddenly went white with embarrassment. He sheepishly left the room; sadly he didn't apologize until much later. Yet more ignorance of my illness, "Do I need a sign on my forehead or something" I thought.

As evening began to descend we all got ready to see a show at the London Palladium. We went to see "*Joseph and the Amazing Technicolor Dreamcoat*"; originally starring Jason Donovan, but his understudy Phillip Schofield had to take over. Once again we boarded an accessible taxi and off we went through the city watching the bright red and white lights flash past. The rain soaked windscreen magnifying the wonderful sights of old London town.

We pulled up near the theatre and made our way to the entrance, a few moments later I was sitting in the dark auditorium. Suddenly very loud music started playing; I could feel it pounding through my whole chest. So began the show. It was an amazing night, the children acting on stage were great, and even though I disliked singing it sounded pretty good to my young ears. Phillip Schofield was excellent in his performance. He really looked the part in the brightly coloured "Dreamcoat".

The palladium looked like a grand stately palace, I felt very special that night. A few short but fantastic hours later the lights came back on and it was all over.

Everyone poured out onto the busy street, my father decided that we should go to "*Garfunkel's*" restaurant. For some reason all I thought they cooked was pizza. I wasn't looking forward to that at all, so I argued with my father for a few minutes. Finally he told me they make other food, and I went along with that. I felt a bit silly being so petty, but I was only eight. We got to the restaurant and had a lovely meal; the waitresses were very good towards us. At dessert my father saw something called a "*French Kiss*" on the menu and asked for it from a waitress, she laughed and so did everyone else. It took me a few years to get the joke. A blissfully innocent child you see (tongue firmly in cheek).

After dinner we took a taxi back to "*The Moat House*" and tiredly went to our room. My mother lifted me into bed and I quickly fell asleep; having enjoyed my wonderful day in London. It is a cherished moment for me, not many people can say they have actually been inside number ten Downing Street to meet the Prime Minister. I ran through my day over and over in my dreams until the first chinks of light blasted through the thin chintz hotel curtains.

Once breakfast was over we all headed over to Piccadilly station to board our train back to the pleasant greenness of Wales. Not long after it pulled away; the hours seemed to quickly fly past. It wasn't long until the signs started turning bilingual between Welsh and English. You always know you're in Wales when you see the sign emblazoned with "*Croeso y Gymru*", welcome to Wales. Thus ended my fabulous wish granted by the "*Starlight Foundation*" to which I'm truly thankful. That small escape from my illness was of welcome relief to the whole family at an extremely difficult time. If anyone else in a similar position gets an opportunity like this I would very much recommend it.

# *Age Nine*

After my ninth birthday the new routine of full time wheelchair user was sinking in slowly; it brings with it a unique perspective to life and can also be extremely hard work. In school things were going well, but afternoon tiredness was really having an impact on my learning. I couldn't take much in and my spelling would become terrible. The best time for me to learn was in the mornings; otherwise I would have been too tired to absorb new information.

I remember having to learn from home one time because of an operation I had on my legs. I had to go to Cardiff Royal Infirmary one early winters' morning. DMD can cause "Contractures". Where ankle, knee, hip and arm joints have shorter muscles connected to them causing bent and deformed limbs; because of the associated Duchenne's muscle cell death. That makes it impossible to completely straighten your arms or legs without causing huge damage and pain. So in an effort to prevent the worst of these effects on my legs, the orthopaedic surgeon who saw me, Mr O'Doherty (a medium built man with very dark hair) said he was going to cut my hip flexors, hamstrings and ankle tendons.

The operation started at nine a.m. and lasted an hour; when I awoke I was very carefully monitored, DMD has many potential surgical complications that could be highly dangerous to the affected person. Care has to be taken especially when anaesthetics are used, if they need to be used certain paralytic substances should be avoided, for example the drug succinylcholine amongst others (many sources including Muscular Dystrophy Canada http://www.muscle. ca and PPMD http://www.parentprojectmd.org). Preferably anaesthetics should be given through the veins instead of orally because this could severely impair breathing possibly leading to death. Please check with your doctor or anaesthetist before any surgery takes place. Also there's a lot of advice from parents to use medical alert bracelets or to use Action Duchenne's A&E file if an affected person becomes unconscious and requires medical attention (PPMD and http://www.actionduchenne.org). After my surgery my legs were both in plaster up to my hips I was in a lot of pain and on a painkiller drip. I had to lie in bed for a few weeks, bored out of my brain. They even made me attend the hospital school, I was a most put out child!

The journey home was very daunting as I couldn't bend my legs. I wouldn't be able to for a few months either. They were in heavy plaster which meant I needed support for them in my wheelchair. My father being an engineer fashioned a wooden tray that went under my seat and stuck out a few feet. My legs rested nicely on top of it. Once inside my adapted VW van, things became interesting to say the least.

The wooden tray couldn't be secured so whenever my father braked it slid forward and my legs would hurt like hell. I'm sure I nearly fell out of my chair a few times, but luckily my mother kept hold of the tray. It was a journey that usually took forty minutes; it felt more like four hundred! Finally we got home and I was so relieved to see my house, to see my sisters and to see my dog. He was a great dog and protective of me; a small terrier with wiry fur. He wasn't a pedigree breed so he was affectionately known by us as a "Liquorice All Sort".

Once inside the house, I was moved onto the settee to rest my legs; they were burning with stabbing pains. I was shown cards and presents from neighbours and friends; that were very entertaining. I felt too unwell to look at them I just wanted the immense pain to be over. During the first week the painkillers weren't touching me at all, eventually I managed to get relief; more by seat positioning than the drugs.

As I mentioned earlier I had home schooling while I was in plaster, it was fun and I felt I learned a lot. A local lady called Jean became my temporary teacher; she was a kind and genuine lady who I got on extremely well with.It wasn't long until my plaster was removed. I was feeling very tender as my father pressed his finger against my ankle, but at least my legs were much straighter now. I then needed intensive physio for a few more weeks, which made my legs burn in agony. Soon it was time to go back to school; I told all my friends where I'd been and what had happened to my legs. Everyone was very curious, and asked how much did it hurt. A hell of a lot I told them!

My daily routine was more complicated after the operation, as I had to use my recently installed hoists far more frequently. There was no more lifting me onto the toilet or into bed. I had to be turned frequently every night, which meant my mother missed out on her much needed sleep. Eventually I had an adjustable bed to make things easier on us all and to give me some independence back. I controlled it myself with a handy little switch.

If I needed the toilet, I'd use a bottle for urination; made especially for that purpose. Going the other way was and still is an awkward process. I'd have my trousers and underwear taken off whilst in the chair; ending up perched precariously on the end of my seat. My mother would then put my sling on and I'm then hoisted over to the toilet. One time I have fallen out of a sling because it was poorly designed, and crumpled up under my body pressure. It flung me to the floor from a few feet in the air; luckily I did no major damage. The whole event shook me up a bit and that sling was quickly thrown out! My current slings are great; very comfortable and grey in colour (not the height of fashion though).

After I've finished my "business" my mother would hoist me up in the air and then wipe me. I have never been able to clean myself up; my mother or school assistants would need to do it. Not only does DMD rob you of your muscles, it likes to rob you of your dignity too. Once wiped; I'm taken back to my chair, dressed and then I'm comfortable again. This process has changed very little since then except for the types of "clothing" I now wear and I have my sling on all day now.

During school time the other children asked me what I did over a recent Christmas break. I said "I went to a Christmas party and saw Father Christmas!" (This was in the days before I settled on my current faith). The kids were interested in my story and especially what present I had. I was given a radio controlled car; I think it was a silver coloured Lamborghini. That really impressed my friends who wished they'd been as fortunate as I had. My father was a member and director of another local charity called "Focus", which put on the Christmas party every year; I went until I was sixteen.

It was always held around the beginning of December. Sadly *Focus* isn't here anymore as it had to be disbanded due to a lack of new memberships. I didn't know at the time, that my uncle occasionally dressed up as Father Christmas. It didn't matter as I had a fabulous time every year. I would talk to all the other children with impairments and we shared a buffet styled meal with crisps and sausages on a stick. It was held in a working men's club, so there was a bar for the thirsty parents. Every year Father Christmas would turn up at about quarter past four. All the children lined up and waited for their name to be called out so they could receive their present. When my name was called I drove to the front of the hall and waited for Father Christmas to fish out a present from his dark green velvet sack. The party continued and would eventually finish by seven in the evening. It was always dark by then in the cold grasp of the night.

A few months later I was given a great opportunity to fly in a helicopter; courtesy of Noel Edmunds' now defunct charity called *"Airborne"*. My father drove me to Bristol; it took us about two hours or so to get there, on a beautiful summers day. A hot air balloon fair was also on at the time; the white helicopter was surrounded by a huge crowd in a large field. We never got to see Noel himself but soon it was my turn to soar above the clouds. My wheelchair bumped its way toward the helicopter over deep viridian green grass; finally in awe I saw the beautiful aircraft up close. I love many different aircraft to this day, sadly I can't fly in them now, but I often play flight simulation games to kind of make up for it. I also met the boxer Barry McGuigan making sure I got an autographed photo along the way.

My father helped lift me in to the helicopter, and I felt really high up, even before my flight. I was clipped into a huge harness. I was also sitting next to another girl who wore a pink outfit and she happened to be quite large. She kept pushing me against the door, which was extremely scary! Suddenly the engine powered up with a thunderous roar and the rotors started whooshing by very swiftly, turning into that familiar black blur. We quickly took off, climbing higher and higher; rising above thin clouds. All the people disappeared into distant dark specks. The helicopter tilted forward and we were off, about to explore the world around us.

The sights were amazing we could see rolling green hills and the whole of Wales in the distance. We headed over the old Severn Bridge, which was glinting brightly in the strong sunshine, like a sleeping grey giant. It was all over so fast, such an anti-climax; I could have hovered up there for hours! A mere ten minutes later we were slowly touching down in the field. I am very grateful to Noel and *Airborne*; that very day sparked an interest in everything that flies.

Once I was back in my chair I received a certificate, which is still displayed in my bedroom today, eventually my father and I had to leave the field. We drove home spotting all the hot air balloons dotted in the cobalt blue sky. A few hours later we got back to our green and pleasant valley watching the sun dive below the mountains. My father used to call the Cynon valley, the sunshine valley. This is quite ironic seeing how it's often raining here! I couldn't wait to tell my mother and sisters about my super fun day in that field in Bristol.

# A Holiday of a Lifetime

One day during summer my sisters and I got some exciting news. We were going to *Disneyland* in Orlando, Florida! What an exciting prospect for a nine year old. My father had to get a loan so we could go; it was extremely worth it though. We had huge smiles on our faces for weeks and weeks. The only downside was not being able to take my electric wheelchair with me. I had to be pushed by my family, losing yet more mobility. I didn't mind so much, it was so important to go on this holiday of a lifetime. It was the only major holiday I've had. I am really glad to have gone there!

Soon the time was upon us to go to Birmingham airport. We set off with luggage in tow very early. My father hired a plush leather seated car to make the journey in. After a long drive (we got lost in the centre of Birmingham, which was interesting to say the least), we pulled up outside the airport. Once my father got back from parking the car, he put our luggage on a trolley and we pushed our way toward the entrance. It was a vast structure, which had many sliding glass doors twinkling in the sunshine. We made our way to the desk and received our boarding passes. We were then told which gate to head too; it was one hell of a long way until we made it. I was pushed in my wheelchair right up to the plane and was transferred into a small metal wheeled chair.

Once inside the jet, I was wheeled to my seat and lifted in to it. Forty minutes later the plane started to taxi toward the runway, my sisters and I were excitedly bouncing in our seats. Suddenly the jet engines roared and we were thundering down the runway until we leapt into air like a graceful aluminium swan. I settled back in my seat and watched the clouds drift by. All the children on board were given pads and pens to draw with. The film showing for the flight was the "*Only Fools and Horses: Miami special*" which we all found tremendously funny.

After eight hours our aluminium swan was getting thirsty, the salty Atlantic was behind us now. Our first stop was in Boston, Maine to refuel. Sadly they cut short "*Only Fools and Horses*" it never came back on after Boston. Finally we were heading to Orlando; it was a few short hours until we got there. I can remember the descent to the airport, it went very smoothly and we touched down with a gentle cushioned thud. We came off the plane last; having to wait for another small wheeled chair to take me out. I felt like some kind of king waiting for my chariot to arrive.

I was reunited with my manual wheelchair inside the terminal building. I was really glad to be in my comfortable seat once again. Next my father had to get our hire car. It took hours to get it sorted; I think we were all frustrated by the end of that ordeal. Finally we were given a huge car; it's true that American cars are massive.

My fathers' next challenge was to find the parking brake; in the UK it's usually between the passenger and drivers' seat. Eventually he found it between the door and the drivers' seat on his left hand side. He mastered the rest of the controls fairly quickly and we pulled away onto the freeway; a beautiful August sunset blazed down on us. The heat was tremendous; we all intensely disliked the ninety percent humidity.

Our hotel was a "Quality Suite," it had a large pool with a refreshment area nearby. I can remember the huge stinging ants nesting in a crack by the pool. Our room was on the third floor, we took a huge glass elevator up there. We all chose our beds; I had to share with Sian; I nearly fell out a few times, lucky there was a sideboard to hold on too. Emma luckily had her own room being a teenager and all. My parents shared the last bed left in the other bedroom. We settled in that night to watch American television, they even had 24 hour weather! We had a *KFC* chicken meal to tide us over. I didn't like the cola as it tasted so different from the UK version.

Every morning started the same; we all piled on to our parents' bed and ate Danish pastries for breakfast. They were delicious and oozed with purple jam. The first week we went to see the famous castle, and sampled the many rides. I remember a huge indoor space themed ride; we went up to the entrance and my father and sisters said how "gentle" it would be (they were joking!). When we got inside however, I was turned away because I wasn't wearing any shoes. My feet had swollen in the Florida heat, so I was unable to wear shoes. My mother and I waited under a plastic palm tree in the mildly cooler shadows until the rest of my family got back; their faces told me it wasn't as gentle as they said when they returned. My father told me how bumpy and rough the ride was a little later. He said it was so dark you didn't know where the next drop was coming from.

We saw most of the attractions that week too. A bear jamboree was my fathers' favourite memory; I liked the monorail at the *EPCOT* centre the best. A funny thing happened to us on the monorail; which meant we went round and round the track three times. The guards who put us on with a special ramp must have forgotten about us! Eventually we were rescued; although it was a lot fun riding in the small cab. I'll never forget the huge spherical museum we saw on our three trips. It reminded me of a giant golf ball on the fairway of life.

Towards the end of the week I think we visited *MGM* studios. I enjoyed being wheeled around the mock film sets; even though the sun was beating down relentlessly. A perfect escape from the heat was to go on the rides with special effects, which gladly involved gallons of cold water! Our last stop was to watch an IMAX movie; it's a huge screen. It was an undersea movie; the fish looked so real and colourful. However they were about ten foot tall; I wouldn't want to meet a goldfish that humungous!

The second week it dawned on me that our time in Florida was nearly over. I would have to go back to the pain and struggles of a life with DMD. I was determined to enjoy myself extra hard. We met up with some family friends who were also in Florida. I liked playing games with their son Steven; we often shared *Game boy* games. He was into *Zelda*; I never really got that game. I was more into puzzles and shoot-em-ups. They were in the first week of a three week holiday. After exchanging stories, we often met up for dinner in a pleasant small café nearby.

A fond memory I have was when Sian and I had our portrait painted by a caricature artist. He gave us enormous heads and tiny bodies, a shark is going to bite my butt and a crocodile is eyeing up Sian. It looks really funny and still hangs in our kitchen. My sister hasn't changed much from her portrait, but I look so much different to mine. I now have a far more rounded and elongated face, which seems like a DMD trait. I dislike my current appearance; in my opinion I don't think I'm attractive at all (more on that later on).

My last memories of our dream holiday was the time spent on the beach, we went to two different places. The first was called "*River Island*;" you needed to get there by boat. The second was called "*Typhoon Lagoon*;" it was an artificial beach a few miles from the sea. I was wheeled onto the beach on *River Island* in a huge yellow buggy that had large wheels; enabling it to float. I did not try that function out, because I never really liked open water. Swimming pools were fine, but the sea was a no go area for me. Now my mini-tracheotomy stops me from swimming altogether (more on that later too).

To exacerbate my dislike of water I remember a bad sea crossing as we left "*River Island*". It was so choppy and a thunderstorm was whipping up frenzy, electric blue lightning sparked everywhere. I've never heard thunder that loud in my life. My heart was pounding and I was extremely scared as the small boat struggled against the waves, it was violently pitching and rolling. Eventually we docked, I was so very relieved. I've hated the sea ever since then.

Sadly our time in Florida was quickly ebbing away and as a last treat we visited a huge mall. It had absolutely everything; it was totally different to the UK shopping centres I've visited. We all bought small items and clothes; it was so large that my parents' were breathing very hard by the time we went back to our car. Once inside the car, we were melting. It got so hot sitting out in the midday sun. Soon the first day of fall came (autumn here) and the humidity dropped a great deal. My mother was the most relieved of us all, the heat really affected her.

A few days passed and our time in Florida really was up. It was time to pack our bags and head back to the airport. We all were very sad and quietly drove the hire car back to the collection point; next to a taxi rank. We trudged and rolled our way to the departure lounge and waited for our flight to be called out. I can remember watching the screen as exotic destinations flashed by in bright red lights. There was Ottawa, Toronto and Quebec, all foreign to me as a nine year old. Eventually we were told to board our assigned plane.

The same wheelchair transfer ritual started all over again. I hoped I'd see my chair again; it was like cutting my legs off. I was plonked into my seat as I felt so tired that night. It wasn't long until our aluminium swan was gracefully lifting us into the Florida air for the very last time. I don't remember the film on the way back, I just contemplated all the great memories I had stored in my head. The hours passed by me, I felt I was in a dreamlike state.

After a quick descent and perfect landing, we taxied to the gate in a matter of minutes. Again we were last off; there seemed to be no rush to this aircraft travel. I was thankfully reunited with my comfortable wheelchair. We pushed our way tiredly over to the luggage carousel. After collecting our various suitcases we trudged and rolled our way out to find the hire car. It was much quicker than on the American end. I was lifted in to the car, next came the luggage then my sisters' and parents'.

The drive home was a very sombre event, no-one said much at all. A few hours later we passed by that famous sign, "Croeso Y Gymru" welcome to Wales. I always feel happy and safe reading this. Not long after we turned the corner past a small church and onto our street. It was crowded with cars like usual, but our spot was still free. My father parked the car, everybody and everything was hauled out quickly.

Soon after we all went to bed to sleep off our tremendous jet lag. Thus ended our holiday of a lifetime; we all have fond memories of our time in Florida. The people were fantastic and extremely kind. The transport system was excellent and wheelchairs were welcome everywhere; so much different than here. It will never ever be forgotten by any of us.

# *Age Ten*

The few months after our Florida adventure were quite painful for my legs in particular. I had a standing frame that was called the 'clickers' by us. It's basically a steel frame that you get tightly secured in; via knee supports and a chest plate. Then you're pulled up into a standing position. It was called the 'clickers' by us because when I swayed left to right it would start the frame "walking" with an unusual clicking noise. The pain was immense after the holiday because we didn't really do my stretches often enough (it was a vacation after all). It was absolute torture standing again in my 'clickers'. My knees were burning; it felt like my ankles were braking. I would plead with my mother to get out of the frame but I had no choice as it was part of my physio regime. It must have been so hard for my mother to see me suffer though the pain; but she knew it had to be done. It was doing me good according to the doctors, I really didn't think so at all!

The theory was that by standing you could prolong breathing function and avoid the worst effects of scoliosis (spinal curvature). In my case I think the jury was most definitely out. I ended up on a ventilator at 16 and I have scoliosis which isn't very good at all and has caused complications (more on that later). I also wonder if it was damaging more muscle and function than it was supposedly saving. The one bit of equipment that did help my feet was my foot splints. I had them from age four to age eleven. They were like half open boots my feet were strapped into. They kept my feet straight and relatively pain free (apart from in the "clickers"). They were mainly worn over night to again combat any ankle contractures I may have been developing.

In school a lot of things were happening. All the kids including me were about to make the transition into secondary school (high school). We were all meant to go to Mountain Ash comprehensive a local school a few miles away. A lady was due to come in to talk to us all about what we could expect. However I couldn't go, the school wasn't accessible to wheelchairs! I was totally gutted not to be going with my friends. DMD was now interfering with my friendships; this is still generally the case today. They (Abertaf School) still made me sit through and listen to the lady from the Comprehensive School.

It was tortuous listening to all the fun that my friends were going to have. When it came to a small question and answer session my hand went up slowly. I asked "What is the point of me being here? I'm not even allowed or able to go!" This was quickly brushed over and she said I'll find a better school. I didn't want a better school; I wanted to be with my friends. The school had been recently refurbished, but they never installed lifts or wheelchair access. The loop hole apparently was that the refurbishment was an extension to the building not a total school rebuild. It felt like a cop-out at the time. All of this meant I had to look elsewhere, which was very daunting for me.

After that ordeal the first secondary school on our list to see, was called Blaengwawr comprehensive, it is located a bit further up the valley. At the time it was not ideal for wheelchairs, a lift hadn't been built yet (it was in the planning stages). Also some classrooms had tight 90 degree entrances, I scraped my arm a lot on my visit. This wasn't really practical for my needs. Another factor against me attending was the hilly nature of the terrain; there were many battery draining slopes and I'd be stuck out in the elements quite a bit. The school was quickly ticked off our list but we still had two left to visit.

The second comprehensive was in Porth, two valleys away from my house. This would have been a long taxi ride for me; I could possibly get extremely tired making the journey. We visited anyway to see if it was viable for my needs. When we got there, we were all impressed with the facilities. It was on reasonably level ground and looked pretty ideal for wheelchairs. It was a very modern looking building with great vending machines full of healthy choices. The one major actor that put us off was the Special Educational Needs coordinator (SENco). She was a very formidable woman who towered over us. When we saw her, she was telling a child off just because he had a dental appointment. This scared me off straight away, because I knew I would need hospital visits myself. Even my father thought she was scary! That school was quickly dismissed by the whole family.

The last school on our list was called St. Cenydd comprehensive, located in Caerphilly. My father and I timed the journey from our house to the school; it took approximately 15 to 20 minutes. This wasn't too bad at all; it meant I didn't need to be up at the crack of dawn! My father turned my adapted van; a white VW through the slightly rusted gates. He drove us up the small hill past a primary school to the main entrance of St. Cenydd, obeying the 5m.p.h. speed limit. He opened the sliding door and raised the lift up to my level. I drove on slowly and he pressed the button to activate it. I was slowly lowered with the predictable squeaky mechanical noise I'd become accustomed too. Driving off the ramp I looked into the bright blue sky taking in the sights, a gentle breeze was tugging at my face.

The entrance had bright white metal doors; I opened the door with a nudge from my wheelchair. Inside the foyer there was a reception desk ahead of us and the main hall was to our left. We were met by St. Cenydd's SENco, a lovely lady called Mrs Hughes. She showed us around the facilities, including the 'Special Needs Unit', the dining hall, the lift and accessible toilets. Everything was well laid out and easy to get too. One downside was the so called 'Lower Block' it was outside and down a steep hill. On a rainy day you'd get very wet indeed. We were assured that not many classes were down there and that the majority were in the main building.

After the tour was over we met up with a man who taught in the "Special Needs Unit" his name was Mr Humphreys. He later became the SENco after Mrs Hughes' retirement. He told us all the activities students could do and showed us the physio room. I thought he was a very jovial man. Next he introduced me to some pupils waiting in their blue sweaters emblazoned with the school logo. The logo was a leaning tower, which was themed from a famous leaning tower on the nearby Caerphilly castle. I saw a girl called Lisa who had surgery when I went to Cardiff royal infirmary. It was good to ask her about the school. I also met another guy with DMD called Mark; he was really positive and loved St. Cenydd. I listened to him intently; he was a role model to me. I was really happy with this school, I was definitely going there! We then said our goodbyes to the staff and children and headed back to the van.

On the way home, I told my parents how much I enjoyed seeing St. Cenydd School. Once we got home I was counting down the days until I could go. I had one last school year at Abertaf to go; one last year to see my friends. We were going our separate ways all too soon. The next day my friends were excitedly asking me about St. Cenydd. I told them about my tour and the staff. I said how much bigger it was than Abertaf. Also that the food smelt very tasty, they even had cheeseburgers! I still had an empty feeling however because I would have to leave all my friends behind no matter what I did.

The winter came and passed quickly and it was time to get a new wheelchair. My first electric chair was becoming too small for me. The new wheelchair was a boring black monstrosity and it was wider than my last one. My father made me a table; it was made of wood and had metal tube to secure it to the chair. It made writing in my chair much easier; although I was a slow writer anyway. I soon got comfortable in this new chair but I was so fed up with the constant equipment entering my life all the time. Just when I had gotten used to a piece of equipment I was measured up for a new item. There's no choice with DMD you either had to change or be in pain from an undersized piece of equipment. Change was constantly thrown at me and I was quite rebellious against it at least in my mind. I knew I needed these things but so hated having to always accept them. I'm still very resistant to change even now.

Soon the summer was fast approaching and my birthday was within touching distance. I always looked forward to getting presents and cards from my family and friends. I was glad my birthday came in summer, as we could easily go out and have fun excursions. We usually went on our summer holiday a few weeks after my birthday. I was going to be another year older, but I never really thought things were going to get harder. I just imagined being the same, that this was all that there was too DMD. Every birthday must have been another terrible reminder for my parents of how little potential time I had left. To me I thought I would go on and on staying the same; not equating what I had learnt about my DMD to me possibly getting worse. I even looked forward to growing older because adults can stay up longer on a school night! Ironically I look back thinking if only I was child again in that blissful ignorance of DMD, carefree, happier and able to play without struggling.

# *Age Eleven*

I had a fun eleventh birthday with lots of presents and money given to me; it was another hot Bastille Day spent with my family. Towards the end of summer term in Abertaf I had to have one final educational test. It was conducted by an educational psychologist to see if I'd be able to do well in a mainstream secondary school. My mother and the school had told him the best time to see me was in the morning when I wasn't so tired because of the DMD. Instead he decided in his great wisdom to come right at the end of the school day.

It was a blazing hot afternoon and I really was ready for a rest, my eyes were very heavy indeed. I couldn't concentrate on the questions he was firing at me in quick succession. He asked maths questions about fractions, I really was hopeless at them. He asked me to work out how much money was on the table, I did fairly well at answering that considering my immense tiredness. Lastly a spelling test, after an hour of his awful questions I was getting over tired and fed up. He was pretty cutting about my attempts to spell the word "eight". In my exhausted and confused state I spelt it 'Aight'.

My mother was very annoyed he put me through all of that. My DMD always tended gave me afternoon tiredness; imagine working hard and writing all day with your body in cement and then taking an examination. I was worn out for the next day and a half after being grilled liked a spy in a baking hot classroom. His ignorance of my needs made our life a lot harder. The cruel remarks about my spelling weighed on my young mind for quite some time too. I thought I was really stupid.

He then had the audacity to write a report to St. Cenydd's SENco to warn them of my "failings", and that I might be better off going to a "special" school. Good old Mrs Hughes was having none of it. She said any extra needs I had would be corrected in St. Cenydd. They had various catch up programs and a small dyslexia class. They were well geared up for my educational needs. She never believed I was as stupid as he insinuated. Everything would be setup by the time I had to go to the secondary School itself in September.

It was now time for us to go on holiday. No holiday would ever be as big as our Florida adventure. We had a good time wherever we went and always stayed in Britain. I can't remember exactly where we went that year. Over the 16 years I was able to have a holiday; we went to various caravan parks and the odd hotel. We went to the golden sands of Weymouth; we ferried to the Isle of Wight and visited the famous tower in Blackpool. We also went to the myriad of beaches in a town called Porthcawl; I wasn't too keen on the beach and my wheelchairs would protest at driving on them. Gritty sandwiches weren't a huge favourite of mine either. I do remember the taste and smells of wonderfully battered fish and chips. I loved the icy cold lollipops and huge glasses of ice cream served in "Joe's place" in Mumbles, Swansea.

I liked to go on day trips away from our main holiday destination to visit museums and other interesting sites. I've seen an airplane museum, train museum and various shopping areas. I took my chair (reluctantly) on a canal barge and on a boat cruising up Lake Ambleside in Lancashire. I saw Alum bay on the Isle of Wight, with its beautiful multi-coloured sands. I also saw a crystal company called Dartington Glass; they had wonderfully cut and etched crystal glasses. However they were well out of our price range! Also we saw a miniature village based upon and situated in Godshill in the southeast of the island.

We were generally lucky with the weather seeing many a cloudless sky. On one occasion we got really unlucky. My parents and I were in a town called Lancaster one hazy day browsing the many shops. Suddenly without much warning heavy rain started to pelt down and a huge storm erupted, my rain protector was shoved over me and we started to race back to the van. Unfortunately we were all soaked through by the time we made it; the drops of water were huge and so cold! About five seconds after we closed the door we were bathed in bright sunshine again. I thought "That's bloody typical!" We all laughed at that and ended up driving back in our underwear! Once back in our hotel everyone was asking why we were a bit damp; it had been sunny there all day. We still laugh about our Lancastrian soaking today and laugh if someone ever mentions a cloudburst!

After our two week holiday we had to get back to the valley life we had briefly left behind. I only had two more weeks before I started St. Cenydd School. To while away the time I enjoyed catching up with Saturday morning television. My mother would occasionally rent out a VHS from the local rental shop, so we could watch films we missed. Sometimes my sisters and I would argue over what watch. We'd do all the normal family argueing over silly little things like clothes and who's turn it was to play on the computer. We would always make up though, I like my sisters and wouldn't change them for the world.

Soon it was September 1995, which meant I had made it to secondary school. My usual school day routine was to be up at quarter past seven in the morning, eat breakfast usually golden brown toast with jam or Nutella and then I'd be whisked upstairs so my mother could dress me. She put on my white polo shirt and then gently put my arms through my new blue sweater, making sure my hands weren't in a painful position. Next I would be hoisted over into my bed and then my legs were lifted into each dark grey trouser leg. My mother would need to very carefully move my legs; I couldn't take pressure on them or to allow them to over bend. Any pain I got from either of those happening could last four or five days. I would have to be rolled over so she could pull the trousers over my underwear. It was tiring get dressed and awfully slow on a cold winters' day. I'm then put back into my chair and my mother checks to see if I'm dressed correctly.

Once I got downstairs via my lift usually by eight. I'd wait for my taxi to pick me up. It was usually a white slightly rusty *Ford Transit* van. The drivers weren't great and hardly spoke to me; although there were one or two drivers I did like. I was often poorly fastened in; my wheelchair would roll around a lot. It was frustrating asking them to correctly secure my chair most days. They got the message after about four years! How I avoided injuries I'll never know; thankfully St. Cenydd wasn't too far away. I got to school between eight thirty and eight forty five before most of the other taxi's showed up.

I'd go next into the special needs unit and I'd often talk to Mr Humphreys. The other kids with disabilities were generally kind towards me. I had a few incidents with other stronger kids forcing my arms into painful positions and poking fun at my surname. It was nothing my mouth couldn't get me out of; I would tell the teachers, so I became known as a "grass!" It kept the bullies away though, so I didn't care.

It was then off to main assembly, the first day I was laughing a lot. I always laughed or giggled if I was nervous. I'd listen intently to any announcements being made though. We never had morning prayers because it was a secular school; even though it was named, rather strangely, after a saint. Once the short assembly was over we all made our way to morning lessons. Talking and chatting as we left the main hall and descended into the main corridors. My favourite lessons in my first year were French (my birthday is on Bastille Day after all), Geography, Art and the Sciences. I never liked studying Mathematics. I was neutral about Music, because all we did there was to make a lot of noise! A short recess was always taken at quarter past ten that lasted 15 minutes; I used to eat a small snack that was until it took me longer than a quarter of hour to eat it!

Our next lessons would take us up to 1 o'clock by which time everyone was starving and itching to get to the dining hall. Originally I had school dinners until I started having stomach aches and general sickness. I switched to a packed lunch which immediately made me feel better. My mother made cool packed lunches with delicious sandwiches. My absolute favourite was tuna and mayo; it had a taste that made me feel like I was back at home. Lunch would be over by quarter to two but the last two lessons always dragged the most; my eyes would go heavy like usual and I'd feel sleepy. Eventually the clock ticked over to three setting off a frenzied stampede to the main entrance. All the disabled kids waited for their taxis by the white front doors. Mine was usually there by the time I'd fought my way through the crowd. I'd drive on the lift and get raised into the transit van. I usually got home by twenty five past three most days. This was how it went for many years; obviously there were exam days, physio visits and other events thrown into the mix as well.

One thing that was constantly changing was my one-to-one carers. Legally as a disabled child with physical needs I needed a one-to-one carer to help me (as set out in my educational statement). At that time there was a team of seven or eight carers employed by St. Cenydd; but with increasing numbers of students they were quickly outnumbered. I definitely needed a one-to-one carer as I was in a wheelchair full time and gradually becoming paralysed because of my DMD. I needed help writing, getting my books out and toileting amongst other things.

However, I rarely ever got fully one-to-one care. It was often patchy and if my particular carer was off ill, there was no replacement. This meant I would have to ask my friends and peers to help carry my wheelchair table (I couldn't drive my chair with it on). I would have to ask them to get my books. I would have no writing help, meaning I'd be well behind the class due to my slowness. This was highly stressful and towards the end of my school life hampered my learning. For any parents whose son needs a one-to-one carer I would recommend asking them if their getting support at the times they need it. Otherwise bring it up with his school's teachers or SENco.

My first one-to-one carer was a dark haired lady from a nearby town. I disliked her at the time, and so did many of my new friends. She always seemed to have a constant attitude problem. For instance when she would need to carry my table, she was always complaining that her shoulder was hurting. The table was light and the distance between classes was small so I couldn't see why it would hurt, I needed my table to write and study from. I had to have it for every class and at lunchtimes.

She complained about her "pain" a lot, even though my muscles were dying in front of her! The final straw for me was when I had a sore throat and fever. I asked if I could go home (colds or chest infections could potentially cause major complications that could lead to death in some cases of DMD like mine) and she was laughing at me. She also decided to tell me "Oh don't get ill Ian, you're my paycheque!" I thought this was highly inappropriate and reckless. I don't know if that one incident had any bearing on her leaving St. Cenydd, but my friends and I were very relieved when she left at the end of the school year.

# *Age Twelve*

My first memories after my twelfth birthday were of the European football finals. Euro '96 really lit a passion for sport in me, I watched England go out whilst sitting in my bed; I felt sad like the players. Obviously Wales are my favourite team but they have never qualified for either a World cup or a European championship in my life so far. I now like all different sports from football to cricket, to F1 to the Olympics and the Paralympics. I think it was around this time that I became a big fan of Manchester United. I was mesmerised by the attacking flair of the red devils. I can remember when players like Beckham, Giggs and the Neville brothers were "young". They are all much older now and near career retirement.

My other passion is rugby; I am a huge supporter of Wales. I watched them play when the six nations championships was just the five nations. I went to the old Cardiff Arms Park to watch Wales play Scotland, unfortunately Scotland won but I really enjoyed the atmosphere and chanting "Wales! Wales! Wales!" Plus I proudly sang the Welsh national anthem, "Mae hen wlad fy nhadau" the land of my fathers. It was amazing listening to the crowd sing bread of heaven in unison. It always fills me with elation and passion hearing it to this day. I have had the immense pleasure of seeing Wales win two six nations' grand slams. I thought I'd never see them win one in my lifetime, so I am really surprised, grateful and very happy they have won two. I saw a few retired players, including Ieuan Evans I'm pretty sure he came to St Cenydd one day. I can definitely remember meeting the mascot for the marching band. The band comes out before Wales play and also performs the anthem. The mascot was a white goat. A well behaved goat too! We all got to stroke him, and saw him in his red match day outfit.

I was still going to muscle clinic; however the appointments were becoming more and more sporadic. Professor Sibert was nearing retirement and I'd seen no replacements coming in to fill his shoes. Eventually muscle clinic ceased to operate and I would never visit there ever again. The orthopaedic surgeon who operated on my legs (I was still checked by him for a few years) recommended I see a spinal consultant too. I thought at the time "Oh no! Now what..." I hated all the changes happening to me. DMD gives you an increased rick of scoliosis and indeed I had developed a curvature of the spine.

Every appointment with the spinal consultant consisted of an x-ray and a meeting. I went to a former hospital in Rhydlafar (near Cardiff) every few months. They needed me to stand but obviously I couldn't get out of my wheelchair. In a compromise my father would have to dismantle the back of my wheelchair. Then the x-ray plate was wedged in against my back. This caused immense pain and a burning sensation as my curved spine was being pushed awkwardly. The x-ray took five

minutes by which time I was practically screaming for
them to take the plate away. I was in agony as it felt like
a nerve was being pinched every time. In the beginning
the x-rays looked fairly normal, but soon I developed
a 10 degree curvature. The bottom of my spine was
starting to look like an umbrella handle! Every now and
then surgery was mooted, but no action was ever taken.

Soon September approached and my usual school day
routine was kicking back into action. The early starts
were a real pain for me and I wouldn't properly come
around until about ten. After the debacle with my
previous carer I was nervous of who was coming next.
A seemingly lovely blonde haired woman was my newest
carer. I've had a long line of carers over the years; they
were fantastic in primary school as far as I can
remember. This newest carer had a child studying at the
school as well. I was fairly happy with her caring and
helping all through that school year.

Academically I was doing very well, with high grades
in most subjects. However I was quite average in
Mathematics but I was improving year on year with
help from my father and another carer. Sadly Art and
Music were dropped in favour of physiotherapy sessions.
I had to keep my muscles in optimum use to slow the
degeneration. I missed Art but it was becoming
increasingly more difficult to move my arms to paint
or do any traditional work. No computer software was
available to me at the time so I had to lose the subject.
I continued drawing small things at home when I wasn't
too tired. I dropped music by choice; I was never
encouraged by the teacher. I couldn't hold any

instruments in my hands because everything was so heavy. I once dabbled with the recorder but I was so terrible at it that I gave up soon after.

The physio sessions lasted usually between thirty to sixty minutes. I would be hoisted onto a hard foam bed and my legs would be carefully stretched along with my arms. These stretches gradually became much harder and far more painful until I could no longer tolerate them. By the end of my school life, all movements preformed on my arms and legs were "passive" i.e. moved around but not really stretched. Stretching now could break bones or rupture ligaments. I had a really nice physiotherapist who listened to my needs; she would visit every now and then. In between her visits my one-to-one carer would do my stretches or passive movements daily.

Getting out of the chair is also a good way to avoid pressure sores. I remember one time getting a terrible sore on my backside; around the coccyx area. My skin gradually broke down due to me getting bigger and my seat cushion becoming ineffective. I had to have a new air cushion (called a *Roho High Profile*) and foam overlay for my bed immediately. I then endured weeks of painful treatment. District nurses cleaned the sore out daily removing pus and dead skin, it was excruciating agony and I'd be screaming out every time. The dressings they used were very strange indeed. One was a yellow plastic covering to heal the worst of the damage. The other was called *Tegaderm* a clear plastic dressing that went directly over the sore area stopping the air getting at it. It also prevented water getting in there too. Eventually I healed up and the pain dissipated. I didn't like the fact that my rear end was on display to all these nurses and talked about at most doctors' visits. I was really happy the pain had gone as I had felt quite ill and uncomfortable with it.

Christmas was soon approaching and I always looked forward to my great aunty and uncle visiting us. Every Christmas Eve they would come by our house at around nine thirty in the evening bearing bags full of presents and stories of the previous year. My sisters and I were always so very excited. My father made drinks for them; my aunty would like *Cinzano* with lemonade in a tall glass and my uncle would have a non alcoholic *Elderflower* wine. I was always intrigued by my uncles' stories about building old style televisions, radio sets and how he was composing a family tree. My aunty would have lots of stories about her career years and the cruise holidays they were going to embark on.

After many hours of catching up they would have to go home. I felt terribly sad to see them leave; I could listen to their stories for days and days. It was always about two in the morning when they left. We were all tired and drowsy at that time and went to bed after wishing everyone 'Merry Christmas'. I could hardly ever get to sleep; the excitement of presents and Christmas dinner was weighing on my mind.

I would generally be up and awake by nine and my sisters and I would nag our parents to let us open our presents! At about ten we all gathered in our living room next to armchairs full of presents. We each had a seat, one for me, one for Sian and one for Emma. I can remember wonderful toys and my games consoles unwrapped in a matter of minutes. My sisters would have dolls, clothes and the latest perfume that girls must have! My mother would get new clothes and small toiletries along with some wine. My father would get anything ranging from pens to books and his favourite Port or wine.

Once the wrappings were cleaned away; usually into a black bin liner (now a recycling bag) we would wait patiently for Christmas dinner. A few hours later after toys and games were played, perfume sprayed and clothes tried on it would be time to assemble around the dining table. It was always laid out perfectly with knives, forks spoons and most importantly Christmas crackers! Next steaming hot plates of turkey, vegetables and stuffing were brought out to the table. Lashings of gravy would be liberally spread around our plates. We would each get a small glass of lemonade or orange juice; my parents or any guests would have a glass of wine. After a quick 'Good Health' toast, we would get a chance to pull our crackers. I could never pull crackers, so my father would help by holding my hand on it and the other person pulled. I always jump when it bangs; I follow my mother for that!

Once the jokes were read out and party hats put on it was time to eat our delicious food. I can remember hot tasty roast potatoes and Yorkshire puddings. The gravy always added an extra taste and helped the turkey go down. It was a purely delightful time. We would discuss all our presents and have a general conversation around the table. Dessert would always be served next; usually creamy gateaux or ice cream.

After dinner we would all be very full and slope off to the living room. Often we would watch television or the odd guest would drop by for a chat. Recently my grand parents come over to play cards. My father chooses the games we play; I can just about hold the cards. I can't handle more than seven playing cards at the same time. We play for small change twenty pence a pop! It was and still is a fun night of laughter and competition. I always want to win, but my grand parents have a lot more experience than me at playing cards. At about ten thirty in the evening my father would take my grand parents home. We would then watch some more Christmas television and have one final toast to the coming New Year. I always enjoyed this festive time, it was a great way to forget about your troubles and get generally excited.

Eventually 1997 came about and again it was time to go back to school. I had two great friends from the disabled unit, one was called Ben and the other was called Jonathan. Ben was around about my age and had Epilepsy; we used to talk about everything sports related. He was into Llanelli Scarlets and Arsenal. I was into Cardiff rugby club and Manchester United. We had a friendly rivalry and could both argue our case feverishly. A few times he came over my house to play *Jonah Lomu Rugby* on my Playstation. It was extremely fun laughing and joking around and talking about the teachers!

Jonathan had Aspergers syndrome which he seemed to cope with very well back then. He had the odd moment but was always very kind to me. We were both into Star Trek and computers. He had an excellent ability to remember every level of any game he ever played. He would 'walkthrough' many games with me all through lunch and break times. I was fascinated by his remarkable memory and perfect diction. I'd known Jonathan for the last few years as he didn't live too far away from me. His parents were very nice too and full of jokes. It was great to see one friendly familiar face in St Cenydd.

In my year group I tried to make friends with the non disabled children but it was difficult 'fitting' in. I couldn't class any of them as my best friend. They were all from the local Caerphilly area and I came from another county. This meant that none of them ever visited my house and because of accessibility issues I couldn't visit theirs'. They were all friendly towards me in an acquaintance sense. It was quite lonely going through school, but the 'special' needs unit was a great place to hang out with like minded people. I did crave a non disabled best friend back then though. I had a few crushes on the girls but I could never bring myself to ask them out. I was certainly never asked out or even looked at as boyfriend material. That was very demoralising but I just tried concentrating on my school work.

My last memory of being twelve was the 1997 general election. I can remember being fascinated by Peter Snow and the swing-o-meter. All the blue Conservative Party icons were being knocked over by the red Labour Party icons. I can also remember the song 'Things can only get better' playing and Tony Blair shaking everybody's hand the next day when he became Prime Minister. I wasn't a huge fan of Labour but it seemed like a seed change was taking place. Not many people in Wales liked the Tories at the time. I was neutral because I had met the previous incumbent Sir John Major. Eventually with Labour getting in, Wales was given its own devolved government a few years later. This meant Wales had its own political process which would hopefully benefit the people directly. I've been interested in politics ever since that time.

# Age Thirteen

I thought "Yes, I've made it! I've beaten that twelve year average". I had made it to my thirteenth birthday. With expert care from my family and some careful monitoring I had survived the averages so far. I felt pretty invincible that day; I felt I could take on the world! Life expectancy is just a number in reality; it doesn't take into account the varying severities of DMD or the care you receive. I had pretty good health care for the first 12 years of my life although some key things that would have helped me were missing.

Corticosteroid treatment is currently offered to slow down degeneration; it improves heart and lung function and helps reduce the risk of developing scoliosis. It is the only stop gap treatment offered to delay progression by a few short but highly beneficial years and is definitely not a cure. It has some severe side effects including but not limited to mood swings, weight gain, stunted growth and problems passing through puberty. Not every affected boy will have all of those effects; if they do however there are endocrinologists who can offer drugs to combat some of the problems. Steroids always need extremely careful monitoring. They are not a perfect solution and do not help every boy with DMD. What they do offer is more time for scientists to find even more effective treatments.

Sadly in the 1990's I was never offered any kind of steroid treatment. I didn't even know they existed, that is until I recently found out through a charity. If it was available then my parents would definitely have given it to me. Now as a twenty five year old I see little point in taking them, due to the fact I have lost so much muscle. I also don't want to suffer the side effects if it doesn't significantly improve my function. There is currently no specialist muscle consultant in Wales to even ask for any treatments. Doctor Sibert had retired years ago and Wales has been in a specialist 'vacuum' ever since then.

Back in summer 1997 I was enjoying the weather on my school holidays. I have one enduring memory of picking blackberries with my father and my uncle Alan. It was a boiling hot day; the sun was glaring down on us. We all took our shirts off and slapped on the sun tan lotion. I led the way trundling along the black tarmac up the hill outside my house. We stopped every now and then by a bush to see if we could find any blackberries. If we did locate some ripe juicy berries my father and uncle would pluck them off into a plastic box I was carrying on my lap. It was great to help out and I liked feeling useful for a change instead of helpless. We would walk and drive around for hours spotting the different cars lining the streets. Eventually we would head for home, while the shadows lengthened across the streets.

Once we got home it was time to cool off with a tall refreshing glass of lemonade. I gave the box full of berries to my mother. She would make blackberry tart with all the berries collected that day. Wonderous smells emanated from the kitchen all through the late afternoon. By the evening the tart would be ready; it looked beautiful draped in golden brown pastry. My mother would each give us a bowl full of blackberry tart drizzled temptingly in thick yellow custard. The blackberries oozed delightful purple juice everywhere. I always savoured the wonderful sweetness set against the savoury crunch of the pastry in my mouth. The warming custard would fill you up just the right amount.

Sadly due to recent eating difficulties I can't eat that now and I really miss the flavour and texture. It's hard thinking back to what I could eat then. I will always have memories of wonderful restaurants and am grateful to have tasted such a vast variety of foods while I could. Losing this pleasure in life was and still is a huge body blow to me; I really hope they find a treatment to help me eat normal food once again. Instead I'm faced with needing a feeding tube but as ever more on that later.

After the holidays it was back to the grind of school. It was an important year in St Cenydd. Year 9 pupils had to choose the subjects they would want to take towards their GCSE's (General Certificate of Secondary Education). You had to choose Maths, Physics, Biology, Chemistry, English literature and English language. Also a short course Religious studies class. Three more classes were required to complete your quota of subjects. After careful deliberation I took Geography, due to my recent high grades and a keen interest. I then selected French, because I had an idea to become an interpreter. Lastly I wanted to try something new so I took Business studies.

I really enjoyed my new subjects and kept up well with my peers. I was finding business studies the most interesting out of all my subjects. The teacher Mr. Jones made the subject fun and he always had funny real world examples of business in action. There was always a chip shop that had a sole trader or was run as a franchise nearby. Often he would say his family ran a huge variety of businesses dotted all through South Wales. These real examples really brought complicated textbook definitions to life. The beauty of business studies is that it often used current news and business practises. It always helped to watch the news or a selection business programmes. Luckily I loved to watch episodes of *Working Lunch* when we had inset days or if I was sick. The BBC news was also quite useful.

Mr Jones would often ask questions about recent events or current stock market trends. On one memorable occasion he asked the class to name some of the worlds' stock markets. No ones hand went up, so excitedly I shouted out one I knew. I couldn't raise my hand, so in order to learn and participate I'd have to shout out like an unruly child. Most teachers were understanding and gave me some leeway in this area. I shouted out "the FTSE", he seemed impressed I knew that and asked me Germany's market. "The DAX" I said confidently, again he was impressed. He asked if I knew Hong Kong's, I said the "Hang Seng". Lastly he asked me for the American market, I said "NASDAQ" which was nearly correct, it is an American stock exchange but not the one he wanted. The correct answer he was looking for was in fact the 'Dow Jones'. It gave me a lot of confidence knowing I was at least good at something. Most of the other students didn't know the names of any stock markets at that time.

However my worse subject was Maths, I was finding it still quite tough. My father helped me if I had any problems with homework. In the class I needed help from my one-to-one carer, to write down any lengthy explanations or any long equations. I would fall way behind if I tried to write it all down myself. Trying to write faster hurt my hands and forearms; it felt like sharp burning pains. The discomfort would make me miss important points the Maths teacher would announce. I also needed glasses around this point as my eyesight was getting quite poor. I just couldn't pick up the yellow marker pen from the back of the Maths classroom. Once I had them I was a lot more confident as I could finally see the equations!

One morning in a busy Maths class there were three students to one carer. It was the blonde haired carer who was statemented as my one-to-one. After 10 minutes of writing instructions from the white board into my school book I was getting tired and my arm was burning with pain. I asked the carer if she could help me finish off some more writing. Unfortunately she was busy working with another student. She told me to wait. I said pleasantly "Ok Miss, that's fine" and waited until she could help me. I thought nothing more about it and continued my usual routine for the day. At two fifty five in the afternoon I was heading towards my taxi and as usual I drove my chair past some fire doors and continued down the corridor. Suddenly I could see Mr. Humphreys calling me over to an office. I wondered what was going on. I was confused and curious all at the same time but I parked my chair by an empty table and looked pensively towards him. A few minutes later he started to tell me what this impromptu meeting was all about.

He proceeded to tell me that he had received a complaint about my attitude and behaviour. He said that my carer told him I was being 'possessive' over her, and wouldn't let her work with the other students in my Maths class. I was blown away by this accusation and began feeling hot, my voice was getting croaky. I whispered out, "I would never do that to a carer, I'm not like that". I was very confused as all I'd asked for was some help from the carer I was statemented to have. I couldn't remember saying anything rude or provocative. I couldn't understand why she made these unfounded allegations against me. I was given a warning to be more respectful towards the staff and to be mindful of other students.

At ten past three I was allowed to go to my taxi. I quickly accelerated out of the office I was upset but getting increasingly angry. I drove toward the van and the driver gave me grief for being late out; however I had more pressing things on my mind. We drove back to my house in silence; I was going over and over the maths lesson in my mind. I couldn't think of anything that was even remotely possessive in my behaviour. I felt utterly dejected as the taxi pulled up to my house; I didn't know whether to cry or to scream. I got lowered down to the tarmac outside my house. I drove up a small ramp to the pavement and proceeded to drive past my back garden around to the rear door.

My mother opened the door and I drove in. I began to tell her what happened but before I could go any further she had something to say. She told me she had a phone call from the school telling her about my supposed bad behaviour. I asked her if I was in trouble. She said no but wondered what I'd said to the carer. I said "I only asked her for some help, Mam". I wondered what my mother had said on the phone so I asked her. She said her answer was "…I can't see why he would be possessive over his carer. He has been supported by many over the years. This seems very silly to me. The only one he's 'possessive' over is his mother, I can't see why you've rung to tell me this…" My mother never believed I had done anything wrong. I certainly knew I'd done nothing wrong.

After twenty minutes of talking to my mother I had calmed down a little. I then carried on with my nightly routine of playing on my Playstation until six o'clock. Then my mother would bring my dinner up for me. Usually I had either lasagne or fish in breadcrumbs with oven chips. After dinner I came downstairs in my lift. I would watch the *BBC* Wales news with my father. After seven I'd either watch prime time television or it was a movie night. Later at nine thirty it would be time for bed. I'd really be ready for sleep by then. Quietly I would settle into my bed and drift off into a deep slumber briefly forgetting DMD and any accusations for a few short hours.

The next day it was back to school. I was nervous; I didn't know how to react towards the carer. Getting angry would get me in real trouble so I'd have to tread carefully even though I had done nothing wrong. I got to the SEN unit at about eight thirty and decided to read an open book on a nearby table. I think it was a page describing decimal places. It kept me occupied while more students filed in. At nine o'clock I headed for my first lesson as there was no assembly that particular day. I waited in the classroom until the teacher showed up. A few minutes later the room was full with students and the teacher was writing on the board. In walked the blonde carer carrying my table. I didn't say a word to her but she could see I was upset. She fitted my table on; I politely asked for my textbook and listened to the teacher. It was a very quiet first period; I had decided that the silent treatment was the way to go.

I hardly spoke to her all day, only asking politely for books or equipment. I didn't want to say anything that she could construe into so called 'possessive' behaviour. I know this seems childish but I felt totally setup. It felt like a typical them and us scenario and a betrayal of my trust. This tense awkward feeling between us lasted a few months. I was always wondering if she was saying more things about me behind my back. If she was late coming to lessons my mind would be racing. I was driving on eggshells riding over thin ice. This was quite stressful on me; I already had enough to deal with. My arms were rapidly weakening and soon I would have to have more help. I didn't want to be worrying about asking for it when the need arose.

During the last third of school term before our summer break in 1998 I was told I had won an award from the school. It was a high attendance award. The prize was a book handed out at an annual event held by the headmaster. The headmaster at the time was a tall quietly spoken man called Mr Eynon. He was always very kind to me; a perfect gentleman in every sense. The teenagers who had won an award had to select their book a few weeks in advance. I choose *Moonrise* by Ben Bova. I am a huge science fiction fan so it very much appealed to me. It mentions nanomachines and I wished they existed; they would certainly be a treatment for my disease. Today's nanomachines are nowhere near capable of curing my disease but who knows what the future holds. I handed in my book to the headmaster a few days later.

The awards ceremony came around quickly. My father drove us to the school on a clear evening. I was excited to be getting an award; it wasn't for rugby or cricket, but high attendance is useful exercise for the grey matter. Once inside the school I was told to wait in the French class along with the other students who were up for an award. It was very crowded in the room, with about thirty to forty teenagers crammed in. I talked to a girl from my class, we didn't say much only asking what each others awards were. Coincidently we were both up for a high attendance award.

Moments later we were told to file into the main hall. I followed behind everyone; my wheels squeaked on the polished floor. After a short drive we entered the hall and saw a large audience of parents, I was becoming increasingly nervous. We all made our way to the front row and 'sat down' in a rehearsed manor. The headmaster came to the front of the stage and greeted everyone from his Lectern. He made a few announcements before the awards ceremony proper could begin.

Eventually he finished his prepared speech and handed the microphone over to the deputy head. The deputy began calling out the names and awards being received. It wasn't too long until he got to the G's. "Ian Griffiths, High Attendance award!" said the deputy. Everyone began clapping while I proceeded to the stage. There was a small ramp setup for me to use. I lined my wheelchair up to the ramp. My front wheels were on their way out so I had tremendous trouble getting over the initial bump. Luckily a student came to my aid. With a few gentle shoves I finally managed to get up the ramp. I felt quite embarrassed as I took a good while getting on the stage. I drove towards the headmaster and parked so that the audience could see me. He placed the book into my free hand and I had a huge smile beaming from my face.

I then headed back towards the ramp. I turned a sharp ninety degree corner and slid down the ramp, my rubber wheels had no purchase whatsoever. I landed with a bump whilst other pupil's names were being called out. I found the gap for my wheelchair and settled in to watch the rest of the evenings' entertainment. I think it was a musical performance produced by some of the other pupils. Soon the time disappeared and all the students were allowed to see their parents. I was very proud of my achievement that fine evening.

As my parents and I made our way back towards the van we were confronted by Mr Humphreys. I was intrigued by this meeting. We exchanged greetings and then he started to speak. He informed me that the blonde haired carer was leaving very soon. My mother asked him where she was going. He said she was going back to college to study. Then my mother proceeded to ask if this was the reason why she had pretended that I had been 'possessive'. No answer was given but that seemed like quite a large coincidence to me. I'll never know the real reason why I was accused. I was glad to be getting a new one-to-one but sad that I'd got in trouble for nothing.

# New Carer Arrives

During the last few weeks of July after my fourteenth birthday, my new carer was due to start. I got into school around the same time as usual and headed for the unit. Once there I saw Mr Humphreys as usual and we discussed either sport or some current news. It was a glorious summers' day, the green grassy bank outside the classroom shone brightly in the baking sun. After watching the majestic white clouds drift lazily by I headed to my first class. I think it was an English lesson. I soon settled down in my usual position in the middle of the room and listened to the teacher outline the plans for our upcoming GCSE exams. They would be upon us in two short school years. We would be having mock examinations to see if we could handle the process at the end of year ten.

Eventually my new carer came into the room carrying my table in hand. She had slightly curly brown hair and a beaming smile. Her name was Mrs Watkins. She was extremely helpful and asked what I needed for the English lesson. She took out my textbook and rectangular pencil case; it was a Jurassic park case. I had scratched the living daylights out of it using a compass. I often fidgeted in class either drawing on my ruler or beating up my pencil case. At break time we proceeded to the unit, she joined all the other carers who needed their coffee fix. I ate nothing because the 15 minute break was over ever so quickly. It was usually a toilet break anyway. Once my carer drunk her coffee I asked politely if she could take me for a pee.

We headed down the corridor to the usual toilet room. It was a freezing cold draughty place at the best of times. It had three cubicles with horrid green doors. It was rare for me to want the toilet in school. When I needed to be hoisted, I never felt comfortable when the carers put me back in my chair. My mother was very good at understanding my positioning guidance. I just couldn't explain things in the same way to any other carer. I usually just waited or held it in unless I really had to go. Going for a pee was easy though, I never need to be hoisted for that. My elasticated trousers and loose underwear helped avoid the need to be moved. The bottle is positioned with my guidance so I don't miss. It's a bit like the old game show *Golden Shot*, up a bit, down a bit and stop!

At ten thirty we headed towards the lift as my next classes before lunch were on the second and third floors respectively. The lift room was a short corridor which housed the elevator. Each student who needed the lift was given a small metal key. My key was always held by my carer because I was and still am unable to raise my arm off my wheelchair control or table. Not even two millimetres. I'd try and move but all my arm would do was tense up painfully. Eventually the lift arrived and we got in. There was just enough room for one wheelchair and one carer or standing student.

We arrived on the second floor and entered the hot corridor. I met up with the rest of my year group and we waited patiently for the teacher. The upper floors housed the Home Economics room, the Geography department, the History department and the Mathematics department. It also housed the library, but I never had enough time in my breaks to visit. I would need help from the carers to get up there. Invariably they were busy so I just missed out on gaining useful information. Thankfully the internet was becoming popular and I could gain insight from that.

I was up there because of Maths and Geography. I found Maths classes really dragged the most. I didn't feel particularly inspired by the teacher but I tried my hardest. Dusty equations and algebra didn't capture my imagination. Geography on the other hand lit up my mind with the complex processes of the Earth. I enjoyed the explosive nature of volcanism. I revelled in the art of meteorology; I could picture myself as a weatherman. The teachers also illuminated the subject with their vivid explanations and carefully selected questions. Eventually the buzzer for lunch would ring out and the usual stampede ensued.

At one o'clock Mrs Watkins and I made our way to lunch. It was a long way from the top floor to the lower block canteen. From the end of year nine till the end of my school life we had to eat in the lower block, so much for not needing to go there often I thought. We had to go outside past the teachers' expensive cars parked at the front of school. Then we headed down a fairly steep incline towards two old rickety double doors. I had to negotiate a small pavement and a two inch lip before I could get inside. The smells of greasy burgers, sweaty egg sandwiches and highly salted fries hit you straight away.

I'd find an empty table near the door next to all the carers and other disabled students. We weren't encouraged to sit by non disabled students I think this was so the carers were able to eat and help us without having to traipse across the room. It felt like we would be inconveniencing them just to have non-disabled friends. The sheep had to stay in the pen so to speak. I didn't much care at the time; I just wanted to eat.

My carer would pass me my red lunchbox. My lunch was usually two tasty sandwiches, a strawberry or vanilla yoghurt, a packet of cheese and onion crisps and a can of *Pepsi Max*. I'd have my hands placed on top of the box. Meaning I could just lean my head carefully towards my sandwiches and take a bite. Increasingly I needed more help as my hands quickly deteriorated. I would need my carer to practically feed me. I'm grateful for the help given to me as I wouldn't have been able to eat otherwise. It felt quite strange for a teenager to be so dependant, at a time when my non disabled peers were craving so much freedom. I felt so different from my peers but I wanted the same things as them.

Soon lunch was over and the next lesson buzzer rang out. We headed to the last lesson of the day. Usually it was Chemistry or Physics. I was really interested in GCSE science and I enjoyed learning about atoms and the speed of light. The phenomena of astral objects and deep space exploration also kept my imagination alive.

After an hour of study I would be exhausted and ready to chill out at home. Mrs Watkins led me outside, and my wheelchair drove reluctantly up the hill. I dodged students and waiting taxis until I found the familiar van that took me home every night. I said my goodbyes to some friends from the unit and told my new carer I'd see her the next day. The van quickly drove off and it wasn't long until we were on the dual carriageway that led home.

Overall I thought my new carer was brilliant. She was kind and always made everyone laugh with her quick wit. She used to talk in my classes and it was funny when a student got in trouble for talking back to her. I was glad to finally get a carer who wasn't condescending toward me and did care about my needs. A few weeks later I was offered to go on a three day trip away at Ogmore by the school. A picturesque area of South Wales near beaches and the river Ogmore located in the Vale of Glamorgan. I was full of trepidation as I had never been on a holiday without my parents before. After a couple of nights deliberating I decided to take the school up on their offer.

# Ogmore Trip

I arrived at school one bright sunny Friday. The school mini-bus was waiting for me; it was already full of luggage and equipment. There were four of us going on the trip, my friend Ben and two other teenagers a girl with Spina Bifida and a deaf girl, followed lastly by me. Mrs Watkins wouldn't be going with us. Instead Mr Humphreys was accompanied by three of the most experienced carers, some of which were former nurses. We all exchanged greetings and wondered what we would see. I boarded the bus last driving on to the metal lift and swiftly reaching the entrance.

Once everyone was seated and wheelchairs clamped down we began our journey. The mini-bus gently rolled off and we headed towards our first destination. We drove to Cardiff bay to visit *TechniQuest* an interactive science centre. After a few hours of fun experimenting with all the interactive games and puzzles we had some lunch at a famous fish and chip shop. The weather was glorious. Hot sunshine washed over everything glinting off many metal surfaces. We posed for photographs by one of the large monuments dotted around the bay while the gentle sea breeze cooled us.

Our second destination for the day was a police facility in the nearby town of Bridgend. After a twenty minute journey meandering through heavy traffic we pulled into a huge grass covered complex. A *Volvo* police car was waiting for us and two police officers were standing by it in their uniforms. We were all in awe as we'd never seen a police car up close before. After we were unloaded off the mini-bus, we were allowed to ask the officers some questions and look all around the car. We were shown the '*Stinger*' used to immobilise fleeing criminals' cars. It had loads of sharp metal spikes embedded in a plastic delivery device that extended out a few metres. It could certainly make a mess of anyone's tyres!

As a last 'treat' we were allowed to listen to the siren. An officer pressed a button and an absolutely huge blast of sound emanated from the police car. You could not hear speech or even thoughts in your mind. We were very relieved when the officer finally flicked the switch to turn it off. For some reason I always laugh when hearing very loud noises, but I soon calmed down. Our last port of call for the day was the police dog kennels and road traffic building. My most enduring memory of the kennels was the nauseating aroma. If you can imagine sour dog food and dog excrement you're getting close. There was no escape; we had to follow our guide and I couldn't even cover my nose with my hand. The dogs were barking wildly which was a little frightening. It really was unpleasant and I'll never forget the smell!

Once passed the kennels we headed toward the road traffic building. It housed a road monitoring system. This was used by the police to keep track of any traffic incidents in the South Wales area. The building had a great air conditioning system; it was so cool and refreshing to be out of the hot sunshine. We were given a tour and had a small question and answer session in front of some large television screens. Mr Humphreys asked a few questions about the technology and the response times of the police. I couldn't think of any questions so I said nothing. I always get shy and speechless when meeting new people for the first time. Finally we all headed back towards the mini-bus on our way to Ogmore.

Our accommodation for the trip was a youth centre temporarily converted for wheelchair use. It was situated by a grassy field and up a slight incline. Portable ramps from St Cenydd were installed over any stair cases and a few mobile hoists were in situ. The first night we all played English pool; the red and yellow balls clacked noisily off each other. I just watched my friends play because I obviously couldn't move my arms. Then we watched television, I was excited to see channel five for the first time! It was in the days before we had digital television.

Before nightfall we were allowed to explore the grassy bank outside. I parked my chair next to a bench and talked to the beautiful deaf girl. She had dusty blonde hair and a really determined attitude. I had learned a bit of sign language over the years in St Cenydd but my failing hands meant I tired easily. I showed her what I knew and she lip read the rest of the time. I was captivated and I think it was then that I had my first proper crush. I just couldn't stop thinking of her all the way through our trip. After a fabulous few hours of talking we all had to go back inside. I can't quite remember if I told her I loved her or if I just thought it. I just couldn't bring myself to ask her out. Whenever I plucked up the courage to talk to her the moment would just pass. She would run off or I got called away. We didn't speak much after that first day so I never knew if she liked me the same way. I was so star struck by her that she filled my mind for a few weeks after our trip. It was my first really vivid memory of a crush.

Soon it was time for bed. I shared the room with Ben who had a bed near the window. Two of the carers helped put my hoist sling on. They would lean me forward and shove the fabric sling down my back. Next my legs would be individually raised and the corresponding 'leg' parts pushed under. The hoist would be rolled over and the sling straps hooked on to the metal crossbar dangling above my head. A 'raise' button would be engaged and I would slowly get lifted out of my chair. Once at the desired height to clear the bed I would be rolled toward it. Slowly I'd be lowered in and my legs moved to avoid over bending them.

Once securely settled under a duvet and in my pyjamas I tried to get some sleep. My pyjamas were put on by the carers. It took awhile to pull everything up as they were unaccustomed to my needs. The last thing I needed was my right arm placed above my head on the pillow. It helped my back with its curvy spine. A few minutes after the light was turned off I could hear the distant rumble of thunder and see bright white flashes of lightning through the curtain. The rumbles and flashes grew into an intense storm that crashed and bashed over the youth centre. Twenty minutes later it eventually passed over. I released my tight grip on the pillow; I really disliked storms.

The next morning bright sunshine pushed through the thin curtains. I had a very disturbed sleep, every two hours my arm or back would ache with a river of tingling barbs clawing inside me. I would need to call out to the carers to help roll me over or move my arm. It was very frustrating being away from my adjustable bed. I probably got five hours sleep when I was used to eight. After I was washed and my trousers and t-shirt put on, it was breakfast time. I chose some toast with a smooth marmalade I'd never tried before. I needed help spreading it on the wholemeal bread and putting the toast in my mouth. Luckily a carer was never too far away. Unfortunately I had the most disgusting orange squash to wash it down with. I really missed the usual fizzy drink I would get at home. The other teenagers had assorted cereals and some toast like I had. We ate pretty much in silence until Mr Humphreys called us over to the television room.

We all filed and wheeled into the room. Mr Humphreys then proceeded to tell us the upcoming days' activities. We would be going to a canal in the Neath valley; about an hours drive from the youth centre. I had been there several times before with the now defunct *Focus* charity so I knew what to expect. We would be riding in a canal barge converted for wheelchair access. It wasn't long until we were rushing past cars in the mini-bus. We drove up many long winding tree lined roads. The sun dappled lanes danced as we drove past. Eventually we pulled up to the canal entrance. After ten minutes of unloading we were finally confronted by a red and green panelled barge. It looked very long and made the usual chugging noises you would expect from a canal craft. A friendly man put a ramp onto the jetty and we all assembled in single file.

The girl with Spina Bifida was loaded on to the barge first. Next Ben and the deaf girl were allowed on. I followed behind the rest. I bumped over the green ramp up to the aft section of the barge. Two metres further ahead was a small hydraulic lift that led into the cabin. I was lowered down and drove over to a table by a big porthole; the barge gently bobbed up and down. The girls were at the front talking to the carers. Ben was quietly gazing out of another porthole. Mr Humphreys talked to the driver signalling our departure. The barges' engine chugged merrily away and we glided down the canal. The green banks slowly moved by and you could see twigs float in the murky waters. It was a very pleasant trip; I talked to the carers about the amazing weather and the glorious journey we were on. After about twenty minutes the barge chugged up to a house on the canal bank. The engine died down to a low hum and we drifted toward a jetty.

The friendly man tied the barge up to a wooden block and lowered the ramp onto the jetty. This time I got off the barge first followed by the girls and Ben. We all explored the house which turned out to be a souvenir shop. There were many gravel paths either leading further down the canal or back towards the car park where the mini bus was. I proceeded to a small playground area to have a quick look just off the gravel path nearest the house. As I was driving over some grass my wheel dropped alarmingly down a large pothole. My wheelchair tipped up very nearly toppling over; my heart raced with adrenaline. I shouted out for some help. Luckily Mr Humphreys saw this happening and grabbed my wheelchair handles just in the nick of time. I was helped back onto the path and warned to be more careful next time. Now I always look at any paths I might happen to be on.

The afternoon dragged on and the shadows started to get ever longer. We all had lunch outside the house sat around creosoted benches; we all had sandwiches and bottled drinks bought from a nearby vendor. I tried some sign language out on the pretty deaf girl; she corrected my silly mistakes as I made them. Finger spelling was just about all I could do then, my hands are too messed up now to even attempt it. Once lunch was over we slowly walked and drove back to the mini-bus. The sun was hidden behind clouds and the day was becoming increasingly hazy. We all said goodbye to the kindly man and prepared for our trip back to the youth centre.

The drive back was oddly quiet; we were all weary after a hot day. I think we were all starting to miss our families. By the time we pulled up to the youth centre gates it had gotten completely cloudy; that was the last time we saw the sunshine. The mini-bus glided to a stop outside the entrance and everyone poured off. I drove my wheelchair through the doors, past the pool table and into the television room. Our last treat for the evening was a movie night. Mr Humphreys had selected a few VHS video's for us to choose. We all settled down with drinks and snacks, I can't remember the movie we watched but I do remember we had great fun. Eventually the movie finished, everyone yawned as the clock ticked over to nine thirty. The girls left first to be helped into bed by the carers, Ben and I talked about sport especially rugby while we waited.

A few minutes later the carers came back to put me into the bed. I drove up the temporary ramps for a few metres, before I came to a hairy downhill section. My wheelchair slid down with a painful squeak echoing behind me. I regained control and headed through the double doors into the large dormitory bedroom. I parked my wheelchair in front of the mobile hoist. The carers followed me in and proceeded to perform the usual sling fitting procedure. Once safely ensconced in my bed, Ben was allowed in the room. He got into his bed and we said goodnight to each other. The carers turned off the lights. I was so tired I instantly fell asleep; dreaming of lazy days drifting on the canal. Sadly my sleep didn't last long, the usual tingling gnawing pain started to fiercely affect my shoulder. I woke up and shouted for some help, the carers came rushing in and I was rolled over into a better position. This kept happening every two hours once again.

By morning I was totally exhausted after my nightly exertions. Thankfully we would be going home in the afternoon and I could sleep in my bed. Before I was hoisted back into my chair, the carers had put on my swimming trunks followed by my clothes. Our activity for that day was a trip to a spa for people with disabilities. Once I was settled in my chair I headed out to the breakfast table. The others were noisily eating their breakfast; spoons and dishes clattered and glasses chinked. I decided to try some cereal with the usual horrid squash to wash it down with. Luckily the milk in my cereal disguised the taste.

Again we were called into the television room to hear the mornings' activities. Mr Humphreys told us about the spa we would be visiting. Our very last treat would be to go to an arcade to play computer games and use some other assorted amusements in a place called Barry Island. This was to be our last day in Ogmore; we were all excited to be seeing our parents later on. After we received our itinerary for the day we were allowed to wait outside the youth centre while our luggage was collected.

The luggage was packed on to the mini-bus by ten, Ben and the deaf girl got in first followed by the girl with Spina Bifida and me. My wheelchair was clamped down behind hers. It was a very foggy dark day. We set off with the headlights on low beam to cut through the murk. The diesel engine grunted as we bumped over the grass surrounding the youth centre. The wheelchairs jerked violently until we got on to smooth tarmac. We followed the road in a different direction this would eventually lead us to the spa.

An hour or so later we pulled up to a very plush modern building sited in a picturesque wooded enclosure. I was unloaded first followed quickly by the others. We were told to be on our best behaviour and to respect the other guests' relaxation. I drove quietly up to the entrance, tinted sliding doors swished open. The interior was coloured in a depressing white and brown scheme. The girls got whisked off to change and Ben and I went to the men's changing rooms. There was a separate room for men in wheelchairs that I was led into by two of the carers. I had the most painful sling put around me that pinched and squashed me all over. I quickly got changed by the carers and was plonked unceremoniously back into my chair. I drove out towards the warm hydrotherapy pool and parked near the pool hoist. I waited a few minutes before Mr Humphreys came along with a member of staff who could operate the hoist.

I was lifted onto the pool hoist by the two of them then swung over the pool. A ratchet system was wound down and I got lowered in with a loud clacking noise. "Ahhhh…" I said as I felt the warm water lap over my cold feet. Mr Humphreys had to hold me upright in the water as I had no balance and could not right myself. If I happened to fall face first he would have to turn me over or I could drown. I was led to the shallow end and bobbed in front of the pool wall. I was holding tightly to the wall so as not to fall. Everyone else was splashing around me and generally having a lot of fun.

We had a short twenty minute stay in the pool but it was over so quickly; I was sad to be leaving the gloriously toasty waters. I was helped back on to the pool hoist and ratcheted up to wheelchair height. I was swung over next to my chair and transferred onto my towel covered seat. Shivering wildly I drove back to the changing room. The carers dried my arms and body before hoisting me onto the changing bed using that uncomfortable sling once again. I was quickly dressed but my backside wasn't dried completely so I ended sitting on wet underwear which wasn't pleasant at all!

Back in my chair I drove towards the mini-bus where Mr Humphreys and everyone else were waiting. I got on the wheelchair lift and was raised into the mini-bus's rear area. My chair and I were quickly clamped and seat belted in behind the girl with Spina Bifida. I talked to Ben about our next destination; we were all very excited. The deaf girl was busily talking to one of the carers and Mr Humphreys. Eventually we were ready to depart. We left the wooded enclosure and the mini-bus roared down the small road.

After passing through very heavy traffic we came up to a sign for Barry Island. It is a seaside resort with a games arcade, a small windswept beach and some shops. Mr Humphreys turned onto a car park and parked the mini-bus facing the sea. The wind was quite strong with a chilly undertone. We put our sweaters on before we set off exploring. Obviously the carers put my sweater on carefully lifting my arms. The lift was deployed and I drove onto its metal grating. I was lowered on to the black tarmac and drove up a slight incline towards my friends. We rushed to the arcade with our change clinking in our hands. I played many electronic games including street fighter and a football game. I challenged Ben to a few games but I don't know who won as we were just having fun. Lastly I remember watching the pretty deaf girl feeding money into one of those machines that pushes change out with small metal flaps.

Unluckily she never won any change to take back home with her.

Quickly our time ran out and before we knew it we were bumping along the road back to school where our parents would be waiting. It was extremely quiet in the mini-bus as we parked at the rear of the school. Our three day trip was over and it would now be time to work a lot harder for our GCSE's. We were unloaded off the mini-bus and trundled our way over to our parents' cars. My van was waiting for me at the main entrance. My father put my bags in the boot and I drove onto the van's lift. I was raised up to the interior and clamped in securely. The drive home was great as I told my father everything that happened on my wonderful mini holiday.

# Mock Examination Year

The autumn started with a routine appointment to see the spinal consultant. I underwent the same process of my father dismantling the wheelchair back and the X-ray plate being wedged in. Again the immense shooting nerve pain erupted from my spine. It was very relieving to have the chair reassembled so I could feel comfortable again. After that my father and I would have to wait one or two hours in a cramped stifling waiting room while the consultant saw patients. Eventually my name was called out. "Ian Griffiths?" inquired a young doctor in a light canary coloured shirt. I asked my father to turn my wheelchair on as I could no longer do so myself. I followed the young doctor into a separate cubicle. My X-ray's were on a light box shinning brightly in the corner. There wasn't much to see as my position during the X-ray was so awkward. The young doctor who was the consultants' registrar started talking to us. He said that my usual consultant would no longer be working at the hospital and a new guy would be taking over soon.

After we were told this my father asked how my spine was and what will be the next step. The registrar proceeded to tell us that my curvature was below a certain threshold level and I wouldn't be needing surgery. Also he mentioned that my wheelchair support wedges would be enough to keep things in check. I was to be discharged from the clinic with immediate effect. At the time I was very relieved not to keep having more uncomfortable X-ray sessions and to be avoiding surgery. However I did not know the precise muscle wasting I would have to endure in the future, we trusted the registrar and consultant. In recent years my spine is much worse; I'm hunched over as my spine bends forward from the middle at the same time it is curved in the small of my back. I am unable to lie completely flat and am often in pain.

I know now with some research from several Muscular Dystrophy organisations that it is standard practise to give spinal fusions for even a ten degree curvature. It is now much too late to offer me surgery as it could potentially kill me. If the Muscle clinic was still running during my fourteenth year they may have spotted the error in not giving me surgery. It is a pretty massive mistake in my opinion as a deformed spine is only going to make my breathing harder. Obviously my weakening muscles will exacerbate any curvature making it worse, no matter what back wedges I used.

As the cold January days approached the pressure in school was growing exponentially. I often had a lot of homework which wore me out. I was allowed to do my work in free periods I had in school. I could barely write anything as my hands tired quickly. Increasingly Mrs Watkins had to write for me as a scribe. I would dictate my answers and she'd write things down word for word. Any long words I would have to spell out as it was my work. If I made any errors they would be mine. I was still enjoying business studies; learning about business structure and diversity. I had to learn to do a balance sheet, luckily calculators were allowed in this lesson. Geography was still keeping me interested with global processes and glaciers. I always marvelled at the slow majestic creep of the ice flow. French was very interesting as our teacher was an actual French lady. She was confused by many of our Welsh sayings and couldn't understand why people put an "X" on letters. She didn't think they meant kisses! She would call them "smacks".

My most vivid teaching memory was in English class. The teacher was a fabulous energetic man called Mr Key. He made English come alive; Shakespearean stories were no longer stuffy impenetrable manuscripts. Romeo and Juliet opened new meaning to age old conundrums of romance and hidden love. Macbeth was the ultimate battle of wills with witches, murder, suicide and neurosis. He was very encouraging towards me and always included me in any discussions. He also sparked an interest in poetry that I've only just rekindled. One afternoon our homework from a previous lesson was to be read out in class. We were told to write a poem about our mornings and what we did at the start of each day. All the class were silent as some students read out their funny attempts at poetry. I was getting increasingly nervous; I find talking in front of people quite hard as I'm often too quiet to be heard across a room.

Mr Key could tell I was uncomfortable and asked if I wanted him to read my offering out. I was very relieved and agreed. I can't remember the whole poem but a few things stick in my mind. I know I mentioned using my big steel lift and how I would wait for my white chariot of a taxi. Mr Key was impressed at the way I described my television. I wrote "...O glorious box shining at me..." In my house we'd call the television the box; he liked the poetic way I explained things.

The class were all impressed by my poetry and I think Mr Key thought it was the most interesting poem of the day. I was very pleased that everyone approved of my efforts even though I couldn't believe it. I always doubt my abilities and am quite modest. I love to try new or different writing styles and techniques. Due to the short length of poems I found writing them less tiring. I dreaded writing essays if my carer wasn't present because of the pain and burning. Now I cannot even hold a pen (incase your wondering I am using an On Screen Keyboard to type this book out; more on that later).

The year 1999 wore on and our mock examinations were rapidly gaining upon us. The teachers were busily telling us how important these exams were. They were to decide what level to enter for our GCSE's. The mock's were setup like proper examinations with set times and absolutely no talking. Around May or June time we had two weeks of examinations. I was a nervous wreck every morning before any exams. I didn't hold up well under pressure, I would worry about doing badly and letting my teachers or parents down. I would often get a rumbling churning sick feeling in the pit of my stomach. I used to take *Imodium* to calm my stomach down. If the pressure got really relentless I often picked up colds or infections. Those really didn't help me and it would take ages to get over things with my DMD.

The first week all the science exams took place along with French and Geography. I found the science exams quite straightforward. Once in the swing of things I would forget about the feelings in my stomach. Most of the questions were multiple choices with simple check boxes and confusingly similar answers. French exams also had an oral element attached to them. We had to traipse up to a very warm room on the top floor, and answer quick fire questions about daily life and conversations all in French of course. Geography was extremely easy for me as I enjoyed the subject immensely. I think I finished that exam early.

The second week Maths, English and Business studies exams came up. I found Maths hard in places, but a lot of the exam dealt with significant numbers and decimal places. I thought I had hit the jackpot as I enjoyed figuring out decimal places. Ironically before the exam I was reading that decimal place booklet I found in the unit. I never knew what was in the mock exam so I was very relieved to see something I recognised. English language dealt with reading short stories and answering questions based on the content. Everything proceeded as normal for the first few stories. The questions were pretty straightforward. Mrs Watkins wrote my answers out and I was careful to use words that I could spell. The last story stunned me as it was about whether or not animal testing should be used to find treatments for incurable diseases.

I obviously feel very strongly in the affirmative in this matter seeing as I have a currently incurable disease. Many upcoming trials and treatments for DMD are tested on mice which provide valuable proof of concept data. Without them the current human clinical trials taking place would never have started. It was quite a stressful part of an exam as it was directly reminding me of my disease. After that strange and quite frankly stressful question it was time to move on to my last mock exam. I was very interested in the business studies paper. Many answers would jump into mind and I could easily explain the processes behind any solutions. I just managed to finish the examination on time. I was allowed twenty five percent extra on top of the exam time, because of my special educational needs as well as needing to dictate my answers.

I was much calmer after finishing the mock examinations. The pressure was off but a different kind of anxiety was gathering in my mind; the anxiety of receiving the results. In a few short weeks I would find out whether or not I'd passed. It was a quiet time for my entire year group during that period. The teachers were still drumming in to us how important our GCSE's were going to be. A bad result was a poor reflection of them apparently. No added pressure there then!

Eventually the weeks slid past and it was results time. I don't remember the exact grades for each subject but a few things stuck in my mind. I did well in all of them and was mightily relieved to have passed. The one most surprising result was in Maths. I achieved a B grade which surprised my teacher and I had done much better than most of the class. The decimal places saved me as I was still struggling with fractions and some algebra equations. My fathers help was invaluable in this field. Maths is a huge part of Mechanical Engineering of which he is now a professor. The results made my upcoming birthday a little sweeter; thankfully DMD wasn't affecting my brain as it has the potential to do in some boys with the disease.

# *Age Fifteen*

My fifteenth birthday was filled with happiness and relief following my positive mock examination results. I received gifts of money and any electronic games I was into at the time. Most Saturday's I would go out with a social services carer and we'd go shopping or to the cinema. I spent my birthday money on a few Playstation games bought in one of my favourite electronics shops in Cardiff.

One entertaining afternoon in August my social services carer Jon drove me to one of the cinemas in the centre of Cardiff. On the way there in my white van we would discuss what I did during the week. Often he would quiz me on the worlds' capital cities or we'd play other verbal games. Mostly we just talked; he was heavily into mountain climbing so had plenty of astonishing stories about mist filled valleys and bleak mountain tops. It was a great but short distraction from the many problems I faced during the course of any week. It was so pleasant not to be talking about my disease but actually using my mind for practical problems.

Once we arrived and presented our tickets, the cashier asked my age for the film. I said "I'm fifteen" confidently but Jon had forgotten this. He said "Oh no I'm sure he's fourteen, you are fourteen aren't you?" I'm quite embarrassed by this and tell the cashier that I was definitely fifteen. After a few tense glances the cashier reluctantly lets us through. As we took our seats Jon says "Oh I never knew you were fifteen ...... ah but you did say a few weeks ago". We both laughed at his unsure memory. I'll never forget the look on the cashiers face, it was priceless! The film went without a hitch and an hour or two later we piled out into the open streets of Cardiff on our way home.

A few weeks later on in September I was called in for a routine wheelchair service review. It was and still is carried out by the 'Artificial Limb and Appliance Centre' (commonly known as ALAC) in Rookwood hospital, Cardiff. The wheelchair I had at the time was getting way to small for me so I had to have it changed. A new bulky black wheelchair called a harrier plus was ordered for me and is still my current chair. I was so against change back then as I didn't really want to keep facing up to DMD. I could see my peers getting new trainers, new clothes, joining new clubs and going on their first dates. All I was looking 'forward' too was a new un-cool adult wheelchair and a constant loss of ability. I didn't want to be different to everyone else my age. I never really discussed these things with anybody but would bottle it up and hope it went away. If I absolutely needed something, like my wheelchair then I would eventually relent to having it. Even though it was ugly my new wheelchair provided me with independence; after all they are my substitute 'legs'.

The harrier plus that I have is an indoor/outdoor electric chair styled in black and made from tubular steel. It has side armrests that taper away from my knees. This was not ideal as it caused my legs to 'flop' outwards awkwardly eventually leading to hip pain. My sister Sian who is into textiles made me two knee supports out of plywood and foam covered in a black fabric. This eased my pain considerably and I'm very pleased they are there. It has one small back wedge to keep me slightly straighter although it has little impact on my scoliosis. I have a headrest to support my head and neck as they grow weaker. I'm now on my second set of batteries, third set of front wheels and second set of footrests, all due to wear and tear. It's been a great servant to me over the past few years.

One extra appliance was offered to me that I absolutely flatly denied. It was called a *Closomat* toilet. It was a huge white monster the size of two conventional toilets. There were several buttons and levers all dotted around its frame. It is supposed to make toileting easier for the immobile user. The idea was that you'd lean either one way or another to activate one of these buttons or levers. This in turn would prompt a metal pipe to come out in the pan and spray water upwards onto an unsuspecting arse! This was totally unnerving to a fifteen year old. I didn't want to have a different toilet to the majority of the world as well as all the other equipment I had.

I had made my mind up to refuse this white behemoth completely. Thinking about things over the next few weeks and months, there were a number of things that would have rendered a *Closomat* useless for me. Firstly I'm hoisted onto a normal toilet at an angle so as to avoid back pain from my scoliosis. This could have meant me leaning on a button inadvertently spraying my behind too early before I'd even begun my 'business'. I have no ability to even lean these days so I'd have to call my mother or carer anyway. Lastly believe me getting sprayed up the rear end does not clean your back passage as good as a wipe from toilet paper. For me avoiding the *Closomat* was a good decision. However if it works for you then please continue to use it!

Back in school and as we progressed into the icy grip of winter every teenager in year eleven had to undergo 'Work Experience'. We each had to pick a place we would like to go inline with one of our subjects. As I was interested in Geography I thought the perfect place to experience work was in the UK *Environment Agency*. They do a vast amount of work varying from flood warnings to some animal conservation. I was extremely excited as the weeks passed until it was time to go to 'work'. Mr Humphreys had sorted out my transport and accessible work tasks were planned well in advance of my visit. I excitedly told all my family and some friends from the unit where I would be going.

As the big work day neared I was called into Mr Humphrey's office. He had a very solemn face as I looked towards him. I knew something was wrong at that point. He had some bad news to deliver. I was devastated by his revelations that I would no longer be going to work with the UK *Environment Agency*. I was told that because of fears over a foot and mouth disease outbreak they would no longer be taking me on. This was a real body blow to me as I had told everyone I would be working there and I was very excited to go. I felt myself get hot and upset but I managed to control myself.

Suddenly I became worried and thought "Where would I be working now? ... I only have two days to pick somewhere!" Before I could inquire, Mr Humphreys told me that my new workplace was to be at the University of Glamorgan in Pontypridd. I would be working on the front desk accompanied by Mrs Watkins as my assistant. It didn't capture my imagination as much as the mystique of the UK *Environment Agency* but I thought I'd have to give it a go anyway. It was just a set back and I had gotten over so much with my DMD that this wasn't much to worry about at all. I was still disappointed but I did get over it and carry on albeit a bit reluctantly.

It started on a crisp Wednesday morning. My taxi dropped me off in front of a plain square concrete building. I met up with Mrs Watkins and we both headed toward the reception desk that would be my base for the next three days. A kindly lady came over with a plastic binder full of extension codes and department names. She explained that my job was to answer the phone and direct people to the relevant department. I was immediately bored by this prospect; how on Earth do receptionists cope!

The first few calls went awfully. I didn't know where to direct people as the binder was incomplete and often the extension codes were wrong. One particular caller was most frustrated that I couldn't him help out. I had explained I was new at this and it was my first day of work experience. He was having none of it and hung up in a huff but not before shouting at me. I was upset that all my calls were disasters so I decided to let Mrs Watkins answer any remaining calls. I couldn't believe how hostile the callers were towards someone trying out work experience. We all got to start somewhere I thought.

In between the calls a lot of time was spent hanging around. I read a newspaper cover to cover and drew a few things on the sports pages. Lunch was a dull affair sat in front of the same table as the phone. My sandwiches were the only bright things to lighten up my day. Delicious tuna and mayonnaise delighted my taste buds. A refreshing soft drink kept me awake in the afternoon. Thank goodness for my mother I thought. Often students would come in leaving the huge front door open. Not only was I bored but I was freezing cold too! I couldn't wait for my taxi to arrive to rescue me from a job I definitely wasn't contemplating.

The three days dragged on laboriously, my brain was as numb as a brass door handle. I was actually looking forward to going back to school! I was really sad that I couldn't go where I intended to work. Answering phones never met up to my expectations at all. I certainly didn't want that kind of job. Those insulting people shouting at me was a complete turn off. Strangely I still find talking on a phone a little disconcerting. My ordeal eventually came to an end and a relaxing weekend beckoned with its many distractions and the salvation of my Playstation.

As the year 2000 came by and the holiday festivities ended it was time to get back to school. The millennium bug never really materialised as was feared by many so-called television 'experts'. I used to watch *Tomorrow's World* frightened out of my wits that the world was coming to an end because this killer computer bug was forecast. I was mightily relieved that the millennium started like any other with fireworks over the river Thames broadcast on the BBC. As my parents drank their champagne I wondered what this new millennium would bring but for the time being all I thought of was my comfortable bed.

One wet day in school I had my weekly physio session with the usual kind physiotherapist. While she did my stretches and passive movements on the hard medical table we would often talk about a myriad of things. On this particular day the topic of breathing came up. She told me that my breathing sounded 'shallow'. I had absolutely no idea what all of this meant; I felt fine and thought my breaths were deep. This went on for a few weeks at every physio session until other topics came up. Nothing was further explained to me about shallow breathing after then so I continued to ignore it.

My mother was told to 'keep an eye' on my breathing, even though we never had a consultant to raise any concerns with. She was never told to actively seek any medical advice. I now know that I should have been carefully monitored but seeing as I had no neuromuscular consultant we were never informed. At the time I thought nothing more of it however unbeknownst to me my breathing muscles were deteriorating quickly. I was losing the ability to cough and it was getting tougher to recover from minor colds. I always thought as a young naïve teenager I wouldn't get any worse and that my DMD was controlled, but you can never take your eyes of this beast of a disease. It stalks you waiting to pounce when you least expect it.

Another of my physiotherapists' favourite therapies was the hydrotherapy pool. The warm water was delightful but the pool was so small that I couldn't really do much exercise in there. We were only allowed twenty minutes of swim time. By the time I got in there and comfortable it would be time to get out again. It did make my legs feel supple and less tight; also the warm water made whatever exercise I did do more beneficial. It is currently a recommended therapy or aid for DMD patients who can tolerate it.

In my schools infinite wisdom I had to sacrifice a class to take these sessions. The death knell landed on my French class. I would miss a double lesson of French every week; it put me well behind my peers. How was I meant to prepare for my GCSE French exams? I thought. It wasn't really practical to cram extra work in at home as you needed to hear how the teacher pronounced things. I was sad that my interpreter ambitions were effectively snuffed out. In hindsight my school and physiotherapy department could have scheduled the swims after school on such an important educational year for me.

My GCSE exams arrived quicker than any of us thought; the months had literally flown by. Again I had the morning ritual of feeling totally sick and my stomach gurgling away. I was still taking the *Imodium* to control things and thankfully before my taxi arrived I felt much more settled. The ride in to school was full of quiet contemplation and going over of potential questions in my mind. I tried not to think of my stomach or I just wouldn't have been able to concentrate. Once in school I had a completely different regime to normal. If I had an afternoon exam I would stay in the unit and pack in a small amount of revision. Even though I had been revising for a few weeks prior, the extra cramming definitely calmed my nerves. I would rather morning examinations as I could get straight into things without building up a high amount of nervousness and stress.

As with my previous mock exams, science was the first subject for us to be tested on. Every exam I took was in one of two small square rooms adjoining the unit. The walls were wafer thin so if another student was in the next small room I would have to whisper my answers to Mrs Watkins. During my exam I would park my wheelchair by a narrow table and Mrs Watkins would squeeze past into a plastic chair by my side. She would slide the question papers in front of me and after some brief contemplation I would slowly dictate my answers. Any difficult or strange scientific words would have to be spelt out by me. This would take some time so I was glad to get twenty five percent extra.

In between exams we had a few hours break again to continue revising or to eat lunch. Students under examination conditions were not allowed to interact so any meals I had were spent either in the unit or the ghastly square room. The four by four rooms were very claustrophobic and had no windows to speak of. At least lunch provided me an escape from all that thinking! I thought tuna fish was great brain food at the time; although I suppose the jury's still out on *Pepsi Max*! I was totally mentally exhausted by the time I got home. My arms were aching from holding question papers all day and my throat felt so dry after dictating. All I managed to do was flick through some television channels and get fed my usual evening meal of battered cod and oven chips. Bed came all too quickly and my nerves would start to play on mind once again. I would worry so much about failure and letting everyone down. Eventually I would force myself to stop thinking, clear my mind and drift off to a restless sleep.

This was my daily examination routine for the next two weeks. I had Biology with its processes and genetics, Physics with its equations and laws followed by Chemistry with its atoms and covalence. English literature tested my essay writing skills or in my case essay dictation. English language again plied me with stories and questions designed to catch you out. Geography made me think hard and fast on glaciation and for some reason tourism. My favourite subject Business studies went exceedingly well and I was confident I knew business structure and working practises.

My worst and feared subject Mathematics arrived sometime near the end of week two. I was very worried about letting my father down after all the valuable help he'd given me over the past years. No amount of *Imodium* or calming techniques could settle my stomach on that day. Compared to the mock examinations there were fewer questions on decimal places so I was sweating a little more. There were questions on Pythagoras theory and coordinates which while I found them challenging weren't that difficult. Luckily fractions were few and far between but algebra was more heavily utilised. I was so relieved when the examination time elapsed. I had little time to rest before my next exam came around. Thankfully it was an easy Religious studies exam that I breezed through with little fuss.

Gradually the final day of examinations arrived and the needle fell upon French. I was dreading the oral element of this exam as I had very little experience of conversational French. Hydrotherapy and my DMD had effectively killed off my French hopes. I struggled to answer the strange Francophone questions and muttered the few words that I did know. It was definitely "C'est difficile" for me. I felt really foolish because I just knew I was failing the oral exam. I hoped to save some pride in the written element. I had to spell out most of the words and phrases to Mrs Watkins or slowly write out things by hand. I finished well into my extra time totally relieved that my GCSE's were finally over.

The weeks leading up to my next birthday were full of days saying goodbye to some friends and class peers who were leaving school after their sixteenth birthdays. Everybody wrote their name on each others arms some on their legs! Not many signed my arms we were never really that close. Strangely I didn't mind one bit and unfortunately I lost contact with most of them. Now I'm a bit sad I and they didn't try harder to be closer best friends. Distance played a big part in that as I never visited or stayed over friends houses. I just made acquaintances and felt like a bit of an outsider.

Also we got a chance to thank teachers who we wouldn't be seeing next year as some of us chose colleges or six form. I was going to really miss my encouraging English teacher Mr Key. I said a quiet goodbye to him and thanked him for being a really great teacher. He said to me that it was a real pleasure teaching me. I felt very happy to make such an impact upon him. He captivated the whole class and made me 'sit up and take notice' of the nuances of the English language. The knowledge that helps with my current poetry and indeed is helping me write this very book. I didn't know that I would have to quickly grow up and face real life and death decisions in the coming years of my life.

# Age Sixteen

It was a sunny clear day sat outside the Bond hotel in Blackpool on the second week of my holidays. I nervously fidgeted with my small silver *Sagem* mobile phone waiting for nine thirty to arrive. As my wristwatch ticked past its destination I dialled St Cenydd's front desk number and nervously awaited a response. After switching on the loudspeaker I got patched through to the receptionist and proceeded to ask for Mr Humphreys. A few minutes later I was connected to his office.

After pleasantries were exchanged I got straight to the point. "...Do you have my ... GCSE results?" I said shakily. He confirmed this and began to read out my results, in the Sciences I passed with C grades, English again C grades, Geography a B grade, Business studies an A grade, Religious studies short course a B grade, Maths a C grade and sadly a D grade in French. I was amazed and extremely elated to have passed the majority of my GCSE's. I was especially pleased to pass Maths; my fathers help had indeed secured me a good solid pass. I knew I did badly in French even before my results and so was unsurprised by the D grade. After the good news was given out I excitedly bade my goodbyes to

Mr Humphreys, who was equally impressed with my efforts.

I switched off the small mobile phone and drove my electric wheelchair through the hotel's double doors. I crossed the battery sapping crimson carpet towards the seats my parents were occupying. I excitedly recited my results about three or four times before I finally calmed down. My parents were very proud of me and offered their sincere congratulations. My father and I had to settle a bet we had made, I would get £5 for every C grade, £10 for every B grade and £15 for any A grades and £5 taken away if I had less than a C grade. I had done very well receiving over £50 and had a beaming smile from ear to ear.

A few days later I was allowed to buy a present for my self. I decided to buy Cricket 2000 for my Playstation as I was really interested in that sport. I couldn't wait to get home to fire up my computer and smash a few sixes! Before then I had one or two days of my holiday remaining. I often read books and filled in crosswords to pass the time. I remember visiting *Morrison's* for the very first time and marvelled at its enormous aisles filled with more than just food. It was totally different to the little shopping centres near Abercynon.

Eventually it was time to drive back to Wales to our home in the green and pleasant Cynon valley. It would usually be a tight squeeze getting into the van with my bed crammed in next to me. I had to take my entire bed because of the scoliosis I had; the usual back pain I suffered precluded me from sleeping on a normal bed.

Our luggage would fit in the extensive boot area and my dismantled mobile hoist ready for transport would be resting on my rear wheels. If we had a smaller vehicle holidaying would have been very difficult if not impossible. I would stay in this position for around six hours while my father swiftly drove us back home. We saw many green farms and rode the cold hard motorways until the familiar sign "Croeso y Gymru", Welcome to Wales was passed. I felt extremely happy to be finally home in what my opinion is a glorious country.

I was glad when we finally arrived home as I could tell all the family my results. I was roundly congratulated and applauded for my efforts. However my sister Sian always insisted that I didn't revise for my exams and winged it. I would laugh but I knew that I had revised quite a bit; granted I didn't really push myself too hard. I didn't really absorb much information by reading highlighted passages over and over again. I liked to do short bursts over various times, it may have seemed like I didn't revise much at all but I did it in my own way. I think I picked up more information in the classroom than I ever did after the fact rereading textbooks. While writing was so hard, it paid dividends to intently listen to anything my teachers would say. This was the key in my opinion to achieving the good grades I eventually got.

Autumn swiftly arrived with its multicoloured leaves and strong winds. It was time for me to join St Cenydd's sixth form. I had decided pretty much instantaneously to go into sixth form after my results came in. On the induction day we had to decide what classes we were going to take. I went for the full allotment of choices a student could have and chose Chemistry, Biology, Geography and Business studies. It was an exciting first day; thinking ahead to our collective unknown futures. I wondered what if any job I might get. However I didn't realise the intensity of work facing me, GCSE to A/S (Advanced Subsidiary) level was an incredibly huge jump I was not prepared for.

After the first week I was already feeling swamped by the amount of homework I was expected to do. It was physically draining on my hands which were much worse this particular year. I couldn't write much at all so my mother often acted as a scribe for me at home. The stress poured on us was almost palpable; I felt terribly worried almost daily. I didn't want to let any of the teachers down or more importantly myself. Mr Humphreys could see how much I was struggling and recommended I drop Biology to take some pressure off myself. I reluctantly agreed but I kind of felt like I was somehow 'stupid' compared to my peers. Obviously I knew I wasn't stupid, although I did feel I was behind everybody else in year twelve. The pressure dropped only marginally but I thought I'd battle on and see how it goes with the three remaining subjects I had. I wondered what more could happen to me, a question I really wish I hadn't asked.

I couldn't get over how difficult Chemistry was; it was so utterly and completely different to the GCSE version. Atoms didn't behave in the same way, gone had the neat concentric circular designs and in their places were complicated P and S diagrams. I was lost in a void of confusion I certainly wasn't used too. We were basically told to unlearn all we were taught from age eleven to age sixteen. Chemistry became a new subject all over again. I just could not get to grips with it as well as also studying Geography and Business studies. I had no means or opportunity to cope with all the extra work, it was impossible to go to the library and at home I needed to rest. I had frequent stressful dreams filled with pure worry.

Another indication of my inability to cope with the pressure was when I sat a routine A/S level Chemistry test. An A/S level is equivalent to half of the UK A level. I thought I had coped quite well with the questions and was hopeful that I might get a D grade. Imagine my surprise and horror when the exam paper dropped in my lap and there was a huge U stamped in dried red ink. U is the worst possible grade to get it means "unclassified", it is worse than a fail! I was immensely embarrassed and felt upset and disgusted with myself. I was obviously not cut out for a life in Chemistry, a lab technician I certainly wasn't.

To compound things even further I was summoned to Mr Humphreys' office to talk about my failure. I was still quite upset and fighting back some tears as he kept asking why I was struggling with Chemistry. I was getting slightly annoyed as I felt it was none of his business, he wasn't even my Chemistry teacher and I told him this. He insisted it was in his interests; although now I suppose I can see he had a point. He was looking out for me, even though like every other teenager I felt I had everything under control.

In the very first few weeks of 2001 I had to drop Chemistry I just didn't have what it takes for that subject. My stress levels dropped off a little more but it didn't last as the Geography and Business studies teachers ramped up the pressure as we neared our end of term exams. I coped quite well with Business studies but the amount of homework seemed ludicrous for someone with ever increasing paralysis. I was starting to feel very weary and lethargic most days; I don't know how other students coped. They were able to eat, write and study all at the same time and I couldn't even do that in my wildest dreams.

Geography was increasingly focusing on activities 'out in the field'. This literally meant expeditions to rivers and mountainsides. One memorable occasion on a trip to the beautifully green Gower peninsula, we were asked to go neck high in a river to take measurements. This was impossible for me and my wheelchair, it definitely wasn't a submarine! As most of the course was increasingly getting physical again I had to drop yet another subject. In my estimation I was about eighty percent paralysed needing increasing amounts of care and support. This meant Duchenne's Muscular Dystrophy was taking away any possible hopes I had with a Geography career. Year twelve life seemed so extremely hard I felt I was nearing a breaking point. I felt so tired and stressed out and I knew I really wasn't coping.

Around April time I can remember a lot of students and staff coming down with all sorts of colds and flu like symptoms. It seemed everywhere I went and in most classrooms many people would be coughing sometimes unintentionally towards me. I never knew how much danger I was in, remember that I was unknowingly losing my cough ability and my breathing muscles were getting increasingly worse. All this was adding pressure to my immune system as well as the year twelve worries and pressures. Inevitably my defences were weakening around me and the point of no return had been passed. This ugly monster called Duchenne Muscular Dystrophy was about to rear its head and bite chunks out of me.

# The Ugly Monster Rears Its Head

The savagery of DMD finally hit in May 2001. On a grey Friday morning I fell ill with what appeared to be a cold. My mother called the doctor out and I was advised to stay home from school and take plenty of fluids and some paracetamol. Also I had to take two spoonfuls a day of a children's antibiotic that was left with us. By the evening I felt absolutely terrible and only managed a few mouthfuls of food. My eyes were watering and my nose was streaming all sorts of disgusting coloured fluids. My chest felt tight and breathing was becoming harder. I was very exhausted by bed time and tried my very hardest to sleep in my adjustable bed.

I had an awful nights sleep however. My lungs felt as if they were being flooded with fluid every half an hour. I would cough and cough and cough but I was far too weak to dislodge any muck from my chest. I had to call my mother to stay with me at my bedside as I was finding breathing so hard. I was getting very frightened and didn't know what was happening to me. The following hours dragged past, all the while I was wide awake and I really didn't notice when the dawn arrived outside.

I kept taking the antibiotics and painkillers but they were just not touching me. On the Saturday I only managed to eat one solitary chip as I just didn't feel like eating whilst battling my lungs to breathe. I remember trying to focus on the television to take my mind off the pain and fright; the snooker world championship was on at the time. I tried hard to concentrate on the little balls fizzing around on the green baize. No matter what I did I could not get comfortable, my voice was becoming increasingly hoarse and less audible. I felt totally breathless and thoroughly exhausted by that evening.

Saturday night was impossible to deal with, whenever I tried to lay down an uncontrollable cough would develop and I'd have to quickly raise my adjustable bed. I was starting to see and hear things that weren't really there, a slight delirium descended upon me. After hours of moving my bed up and down I could not tolerate any more so yet again I had to wake my mother. At about four in morning I was moved back into my chair which I rode into the lounge, my mother stayed with me trying out all sorts of homemade remedies. I tried hot honey and lemon drinks, going under a towel over some steam and various cold and flu remedies. Sadly none of these were working on my symptoms.

I was so tired I could hardly open my eyes on Sunday morning. No matter how much I tried to rest or sleep my chest would erupt into a huge coughing fit. All I could do was concentrate on my breathing; I could feel all the fluid moving up and down my windpipe. Every cough would make the sticky secretions clog in my throat but I just managed to dislodge them and breathe in gulps of cool air my body was craving. It was tremendously scary for that split second where I couldn't breathe; my heart would pound away at a tremendous rate of knots. I knew I was in serious trouble as the evening fell. No food and hardly any drink were consumed by me at all on that cold grey Sunday, exhaustion and dehydration were only increasing my delirium.

As bed time neared I felt increasingly upset and weary and was often in tears. I felt like I was drowning in my chest fluids. My cough was getting so weak as to make it barely audible. My mother put me in my bed but a short hour later I was calling out again. My lungs were on fire with pain; even lying at a slight angle would set off my ineffective cough. I asked my mother to take me back to the lounge. Once there for some reason I decided to be hoisted onto one of the lounge armchairs. My mother used my mobile hoist and gently placed me in the middle of the chair, I rested my weary head on the sling strap which was still attached to the hoist. Trying to calm my feelings and emotions my mother switched on the television. I remember vividly watching a football show called 'Champions' League weekly'. I tried to listen but it was so hard moving my chest in and out that I don't remember many words. All I remember is watching glossy white footballs floating sinuously through the black chilled night air.

My strange odyssey of watching television whilst attached to a cold white hoist continued into the morning. My father woke up at about eight he took one look at my ill and increasingly frail body and decided that I should seek medical aid at the hospital. He had seen me quickly deteriorate over the past four days and became significantly concerned at my continuing distress. I totally agreed that I needed to seek professional medical help. My chest was very noisy and at that moment it felt as if there was a perfect storm brewing in my lungs. My mother put me back in the wheelchair and I shivered profusely as she covered me in fleece blankets; I was only wearing a tee shirt at the time as I was too sick to roll over on my bed to get dressed.

Whilst my mother was securing me into the wheelchair my father rang the only medical professional who knew about me. It turned out to be none other than Professor Sibert who was once in charge of the now defunct muscle clinic. My father got through to his house and proceeded to ask where they should take me for treatment, my father sounded so very worried whilst he talked to the professor. It was recommended that we go to Llandough (Llan-doc) hospital in Penarth. After he hung up the phone my father quickly hobbled over to our van and brought it round to the front of the house. He was hobbling because he had a small cast on his leg. A few weeks earlier he had an unfortunate accident falling from a ladder fracturing a bone in his foot. He was fine although shaken up a little bit.

Meanwhile my mother and I proceeded to go around the back of my house towards the side entrance that led onto the street. As I trundled slowly onto the pavement I could see the van's lift awaiting my arrival. I drove on and my father raised me up to floor level where I carefully backed into the van. He then proceeded to fasten my wheelchair in with clamps, brakes and a red safety belt that went under my arms. I was still shivering under the thick fleece blankets swathed around me. I managed to cough a little and brought up some disgusting greenish-brown mucus into a piece of kitchen towel that my mother held in front of me. I was crying with the fire burning deep inside my lungs, I just wanted to be better and breathing easily. I wondered why all this was happening to me and what had I done to deserve it!

My father started the engine and quickly accelerated towards the end of our street. I remember the journey quite well as we still go there now. We joined the dual carriage way and headed toward a large roundabout near Cardiff. Next we would join a motorway and pass a few junctions until we reached a turn off. At the turn off we would be confronted by another large roundabout, we took the first turn onto the most uncomfortable road that you could imagine. It was paved in a concrete that rumbled and bounced the van as we travelled along its surface. It shook my painful struggling chest for a few miles but I didn't really care; I knew we were going to a place that could help. Moments later we came to yet another turn off and roundabout section, this time we took the second turning onto a straight road. We passed a pub and went through traffic lights shining brightly in green. A few minutes later we turned by yet another pub up a short hill and through the gates of Llandough hospital. Overall this journey can take anywhere from forty minutes to one and a half hours depending on traffic conditions.

We pulled up outside the children's ward entrance, it had brightly coloured murals featuring clowns and flowers on its windows. My father quickly brought the van's fold away lift up to floor level I then slowly edged on to its rough metal surface. I was lowered down to pavement level with the familiar squeaks and rattles that were unique to this lift. I felt relieved, surely the stronger antibiotics I would be given would kick in and the excess fluids would quickly drain away. I was led toward two large double doors which I proceeded to go through. I immediately noticed how much warmer the corridor was once safely inside.

I was met by two friendly nurses who pointed me in the direction of a side room that had been reserved for me. I wearily drove my wheelchair into the hot room and parked in front of a small children's hoist. I started coughing, my ineffective chest muscles working overtime but the nurses swiftly told me "Please don't cough! ... Try not to cough!" I had no idea why but I found it hard not to as my lungs were burning in agony. I suppose they were trying to stop the spread of whatever illness I had. Next I had my own sling taken off from around me under protest. In its place a small totally cumbersome purple sling was shoved hastily around me. The nurses then attached it to the children's hoist and started to raise me up.

It was very uncomfortable as I felt I was being crushed which only exacerbated my breathing difficulties. At the same time I was sure I was sliding out of the sling. I screamed something along the lines of "Help! I'm slipping ...... be quick or I'll fall out! Please!" My heart started yammering with the fright. This prompted the nurses to quickly shove the hoist over the bed and I just got on it in time. The sling was removed and I weakly coughed for about ten minutes, the nurses again admonished me for doing so. Eventually I managed to control my coughing by dribbling out of my mouth onto a paper towel. I was sweating more and more by this time and felt totally exhausted.

Outside my room on the children's ward my parents were talking to one of the doctors who worked up on intensive care. His name was Dr Hebden and he suggested that I may need something called a mini tracheotomy put in my neck. It would enable the excess secretions to be sucked away seeing as my weak cough wasn't currently clearing me. My parents didn't know exactly what to do so waited to see if the drugs they were pumping into me had any effect. If that didn't work the doctors were free to try any means to make me feel better. Having no sleep for four days as well as my burning chest pain, had put me in a very confused and delirious state which the doctors wanted to rectify.

Meanwhile I was being poked and prodded by the nurses, they asked for any medical history I had. Obviously I told them about suffering from "Duchenne's Muscular Dystrophy". I also mentioned having mild asthma as well as telling them what had been going on over the past few days. Intravenous drips' were inserted into either arm with extreme difficulty. I have contractures at my elbow so straightening them is impossible as they are permanently bent at forty five degrees. All drips and blood taking are done on my forearms using very thin or "butterfly" needles. I had no idea what they were pumping into my bloodstream. My lungs were still hurting and I felt gravely ill, I was getting impatient because I wanted some relief from this ghastly sickness.

The hours dragged on slowly and painfully I didn't know how they were going to improve my situation. My uncle Alan popped in to see how I was doing and to see if I was alright in the afternoon. At the time and while my family were watching a nurse called Helen brought in a long thin tube and explained that it was a suction catheter. She was planning on feeding it down my nose passed the back of my throat and in to my windpipe to try to clear the mucus from my lungs.

She attached the tube to the hospital suction and began feeding it down my nose. It was so painful; it felt like it was cutting all my air off. I could feel it snaking its way around the back of my throat and sliding through mucus membranes into my windpipe. The secretions were violently moving up and down my trachea and occasionally they would get stuck stubbornly, I just managed to move the blockage with a cough in time which increased the burning pain panging in my chest. She started the suction but after a few attempts she wasn't getting anything up at all it was too thick, my eyes started watering profusely. My ineffective cough started up and it was extremely hard to control.

Helen then removed the catheter to check on my progress. Two or three minutes later I turn to look at my uncle when out of nowhere another cough erupted. I felt a huge plug of mucus move in my trachea I tried to cough it out but it got firmly stuck. I tried desperately to breathe my lungs burst into pain as they ached for some life giving air. I tried harder and harder to breathe and the pain intensified beyond anything I knew. My heart pounded so loudly in my ears. I was drowning in a pool of my own fluid secretions. I knew something bad was going happen. Suddenly my eyes rolled back and everything went black at the same time my body slumped dangerously back. Was this the end of me, I thought I would surely die. I fell unconscious and to this day don't remember what happened next.

My mother has recently filled in the difficult blanks for me. Helen immediately pressed a big red crash alarm button and all hell tore loose. Lots of staff came running in to help out and to clear the area. Helen was saying "Stay with me, Ian, Stay with me!" I was laid on my back and the bed quickly wheeled out toward a nearby lift. My parents were told that the nurses were taking me to intensive care. My mother asked if she could go with me as she had been there with me from the beginning of my life. The nurses said she would have to wait outside ICU while they worked on me. She felt totally helpless as they wheeled my bed away. She was very upset and tearful overcome with the shock of seeing me collapse. I really can't imagine what it's like for a parent to go through any of this.

On the way there a doctor called Sian preformed an emergency tracheotomy on me to insert the previously mentioned mini tracheotomy. A hole just under a centimetre in diameter is cut into my neck with a scalpel and a curved four inch long plastic tube is fed into my throat through the aforementioned hole. Unbeknownst to me blood poured everywhere, over my neck, over the bed and the sheets. The tube allows easy access for the thin suction catheters that Helen used earlier. The mucus plug was eventually removed with extensive suctioning but I was still unconscious. After a short journey by lift to the second floor I was wheeled toward the intensive care entrance.

The bed with my frail unconscious body burst through the intensive care doors and I was wheeled next to another. I was quickly transferred onto the specialised medical bed and assessed by doctor Hebden. It was decided that I needed to be put on a ventilator. They chose something called a *Nippy 1* ventilator. It is a 'NIPPV' machine and that either stands for a Non Invasive Positive Pressure Ventilator or a Nasal Intermittent Positive Pressure Ventilator. A full face mask was tightly secured onto my face to eliminate any air leaks. A pipe is then attached to the machine and then to the mask. The machine is then set to the correct pressure and air volume settings. Finally it is turned on and immediately begins to pump air into the mask under pressure where it inflates the lungs. It cycles between pumping air in and stopping allowing my exhalation. Oxygen was also added to the mix of gasses pushed in to my lungs to ease my suffering.

A few minutes after the ventilator was switched on I regained consciousness. I saw through bleary and short sighted eyes what looked like doctor Hebden. I was overcome with emotion as the deep cooling breaths pumped in their delightful life sustaining air. I keep repeating myself over and over between breaths to doctor Hebden, "....Thank you for saving ... my life! ... Thank you for saving ... my life! ..." He couldn't understand me as the mask made my voice sound extremely muffled and again barely audible. I quickly felt the tiredness pounce on me as if it were a leopard and I could no longer keep my eyes open.

I slept for hours and every now and then a nurse would put another suction catheter down the mini tracheotomy to clear my airways. A cocktail of drugs was administered via a cannula inserted into my vein. I also had an arterial line put in too; this was used for blood taking. I had blood taken every few hours by a few a very kind phlebotomists. It was quite noisy in the intensive care unit various pings and bleeps could be heard wailing away in the distance. Very strong antibiotics were given to me but these only added to my tiredness.

My family were allowed to visit me in intensive care shortly after I was stabilised. I was so very relieved to see them standing in front of me. I felt as if the doctors had given me a second chance at life. Sian was there and I tried to talk to her but again the mask muffled my voice. Suddenly Sian went very white and had to quickly leave my bedside. The sight of a copious amount of dried blood on my neck from the mini tracheotomy had scared her a bit. She doesn't like the sight of blood whatsoever. I hadn't realised my neck was drenched in blood until a few days later.

The cocktail of drugs was making me feel extremely lethargic. The night flew by while I was on the life supporting ventilator. I remember the next morning as the nurses rolled me over to change my blood stained bed clothes that the ventilator pipe fell out. Suddenly and unexpectedly I had to breathe for my self, quickly my heart started thumping and I could feel that burning sensation in my lungs again. I tried to scream out but the mask and my newly weakened lungs made me produce a tiny squeak. Luckily the Nippy wailed out its alarm and I was quickly reunited with the cool pressurised air that I was recently accustomed too. I had become totally reliant on a machine to breathe. It was an extremely claustrophobic feeling indeed, as the world closed in around me.

In the afternoon a nurse who took care of me when I was first admitted came to visit. We were talking well I was writing on a pad placed under my hand while the nurse talked. It was very comforting communicating with another human. Sadly while he was talking I was suddenly overcome by a wave of tiredness and quickly fell asleep. An hour later I awoke to the sound of the nurse talking again, I was very confused and thought I'd slept for the whole night. I asked the nurse what day it was but he said it was the same day. I did not know where I was and wondered what these drugs were doing to me. I felt in a permanent haze barely able to keep my eyes open. Often I would unexpectedly fall asleep for a few minutes at a time. Missing out on four days sleep had badly affected my body's natural rhythm.

At the evening visiting period my mother, father and eldest sister Emma came to see me. Emma had driven a long distance from her very first teaching job in Essex. Unusually the first thing I asked in my confused state was "... Where's Ceri? ..." Ceri was her long term boyfriend and eventual husband. I had totally forgotten she had driven all of those miles from her first job. I also forgot that Ceri was still in University at the coastal town of Aberystwyth in North West Wales. My mother explained things for me and I suddenly realised my error, I turned to Emma and said that I was sorry. We laughed it off but I certainly was looking forward to the fuzz clearing in my mind. All too quickly it was time for my family to leave me in the capable hands of the intensive care nurses.

On the third day of my stay in intensive care Professor Sibert came to visit me. I found out that he wasn't exactly happy I was being ventilated and didn't believe I should be on the *Nippy*. In my opinion this would have meant only one thing that being my death! I'm such a positive person that giving up and dying never entered my mind at all. The next thing I did was to write on a pad of paper my mother held under my arm. In an emotionally charged moment and through many tears I scrawled in black ink "I'm too Young to Die" which my mother read out for me to the professor. He went very quiet and seemed satisfied that I had made my mind up for myself. He left shortly afterward breezing through the pressurised intensive care doors. That was the last time I ever remember seeing him.

In the afternoon the nurses and doctor Hebden had their usual patient meeting about me. They were quite concerned that my oxygen saturations were not rising above eighty percent. All sorts of drastic interventions were being discussed such as the need for permanent oxygen to be used or to start me on a more invasive ventilator. I was hoping for more time as maybe my lungs would recover. Thankfully the nurses and doctor Hebden decided to let another night go by to see if things improved. I was relieved as I settled down in the bed for another night on the life preserving ventilator. It would force air in every two seconds then cut out for a further two seconds while my tender and achy lungs expelled the cool gasses.

A lot of people rang to check on my condition including Mr Humphreys. He often rang during the day; a nurse would come to my bedside to inform me. I could only acknowledge with a muffled gurgle. My parents and family relatives all rang and it made me feel reassured that everyone was thinking about me. It was an incredibly cold and lonely place at times. However I didn't have much time to think about that as I fought for my life. I'm not sure of the exact timing of this next moment but I do remember that it was frightening. It was a terrible reminder of where I was.

I was facing a patient across the room from me in another specialised bed when suddenly it looked like many fuses had blown. You could see actual smoke rising from the equipment and to compound the issue their bed blew a fuse too and suddenly fell back violently. The nurses all ran over to assist the poor patient and I was very frightened upon seeing all of this. I wondered if the patient was alright and asked one of the kind nurses once she was free. I was told that the person had been extremely ill for awhile and would very likely die in the next few days (which did sadly happen). The bed incident had nothing to do with her death however.

Intensive care is an extremely scary place for a sixteen year old; I had a very uneasy sleep that night.

The next day was crucial for me; would I require more intensive treatment or permanent oxygen therapy. After a nervy morning the doctors were finally happy with my oxygen saturations. They had risen considerably overnight so much so that the doctors were keen to wean me off the ventilator. I was very nervous about this as I had become used to the methodical mechanical action of the machine. A very encouraging nurse who reminded me of Elvis coaxed me off the mask with the offer of some cereal. I had been fed via a tube in my groin for the previous few days while I was being ventilated. After a few panicky moments gasping for air I managed to settle down into a steady rhythm of breathing. I was free at last and could finally talk to the nurses.

However there was one last sting in the tail as I overheard a doctor describe me as obese while I was fighting for my life. I thought this was a cruel thing to say to someone with a terminal illness. I was only at worst a touch overweight but nonetheless I was later put on diet pills. If that doctor had realised what Duchenne's was capable of they would never have put me on them. My weakening throat muscles would only make eating much harder in the coming years. Depleting my energy reserves would certainly not be good for my general wellbeing. All of this will come to light further on in this book.

After coming off the ventilator the slow start of my recovery from what I later discovered was bi-lateral bronchopneumonia could begin. Over the next three days I was only going on the ventilator at nights and my lungs felt much better. By the end of the week I was said to be "too well for ICU". I was reunited with my mother back on the children's ward. I was excited to see other people and not be surrounded by monitoring equipment beeping and clanging away. It was immensely pleasurable to be reunited with my wheelchair. I could move around avoiding going stir crazy seeing that same ceiling tile day in day out.

The only downside was my difficulty in wanting to use the *Nippy* at night. Now that I could breathe in the day I thought that I didn't need to use it at all. My breathing muscles were damaged severely after the pneumonia so I definitely needed nightly ventilation. I had so much trouble feeling locked in to the mask and I didn't feel like a normal sixteen year old boy. A big stumbling point was the damage on the bridge of my nose; this caused me immense pain and it often bled. In the rush to get me on the ventilator I was given a mask that was too small for my face which meant the plastic had dug into my nose. Also the high pressure air would make the mask dig in even further. Luckily a bit of foam and a plaster would take some pressure off. Every night I would argue to come off the ventilator after only four hours use. Eventually I got used to the idea as I felt so much better the morning after. It was extremely difficult getting accustomed to something so alien for me.

Quickly the second week on the children's ward came to pass. It was nearing the time to be leaving hospital but not after one final scare. After eating some chicken nuggets I started to feel very ill one afternoon. My heart felt like it was fluttering away and I was bathed in a layer of cold sweat. The registrar on duty hastily arranged an ECG on my heart. I even had to have an ultrasound preformed. I remember the hand held monitor sliding slowly through the cold gel on my chest as the operator typed things into the machine. I was nervous as the operator made strange faces while checking my heart. Eventually and without offering any explanations the test was over and the operator left. The doctor who was monitoring me on the children's ward never said what the results were. I felt much better by the evening but I had no idea what just happened to me. I was strangely given a diuretic tablet to take but I wasn't sure why as no further explanation had been given.

The last thing to be done before I could go home was to remove the mini tracheotomy from my neck. Once it was carefully slid out of the hole in my throat a wad of gauze was taped over it. The wound healed incredibly quickly and by the next day you couldn't tell that I had a tracheotomy there. I felt much happier now that my neck looked human again. My mother could finally clean all the dried blood that caked my skin. The doctors were happy that my cough was sufficient but it could get worse as no one really knew what to expect. I was advised to do some breathing exercises, such as 'huffing' if I felt any secretions building up. Also my mother was advised to 'tap' my chest by the physiotherapists who visited me everyday.

At last in an excited moment I was finally allowed to leave the hospital. I drove my wheelchair quickly through the corridor toward the nurses' station. I thanked all the nurses' present and my mother gave them all a tin of quality street chocolates. I was extremely grateful they saved my life and rescued me from the clutches of pneumonia. After that I proceeded to the front doors to get in the van waiting outside for me. My father once again activated the lift and I backed in feeling much brighter. I thought this was the end of my problems breathing and again somewhat naively that DMD couldn't possibly get any worse. I still despised the fact that this disease was robbing me of so much, however my positive and determined attitude just kept me going. We slowly drove out of the hospital obeying the five miles per hour speed limit. We then made the same journey home that we would make unknowingly time and again in the coming years.

# Age Seventeen

During the weeks following my seventeenth birthday I felt like I was wiser beyond my years. On our last ever holiday in Blackpool I was often thinking of the future. I wondered what it would be like and what my life had in store for me. I was increasingly worried about hygiene and germs after that horrific episode in intensive care. I could 'see' them everywhere and would often complain at people including my mother to wash their hands. I was so apprehensive that one stray cough or one slightly dusty surface would immediately make me ill again. I didn't want to go back to the hospital I wanted to be as strong and as 'normal' in a breathing sense as every other seventeen year old boy.

Given all my worries I spent a lot of my holiday cooped up in the medium sized hotel room we were staying in. To pass the time I bought the newly released *Playstation 2* from a retailer near the grand tower that majestically overlooked Blackpool. It was my only escape from thinking about all the possible bacteria that could make me ill given the chance. The first game I bought was an energetic rugby game which had in it my favourite and much loved commentator; the now sadly departed Bill McLaren. I would be on that game for hours usually during the so-called 'entertainment' provided by the hotel. It was either Alf and his organ singing songs I'd never heard of or playing a game I loved on a brand new games console. I know which one I preferred and in the end there was no contest, the game always won!

I was often thinking and worrying about my career prospects; would I really have anything to look forward too. I knew and came to realise after my near death experience that my DMD had the potential to get much worse and much nastier. School would be fast approaching and most of my peers and friends had to choose their potential universities. I felt so unsure about my future over that summer, with increased paralysis inevitable and possible breathing difficulties. I couldn't think of a career I could do with all of these impairments piling up on top of me. I did feel a change was coming but I didn't know what was going to happen. It was a niggling thought bubbling away in the back of my mind quite a lot.

In September 2001 I came across a change that I definitely wasn't expecting. It was a gloriously warm day with a cobalt blue sky and a low prickly hot sun. Outside the physio room beside the ramp leading back into the building I was talking to nice girl wearing a long navy blue skirt and her sixth form sweater. I had known her for a good few years but we never really had a proper conversation. She was a very pleasant girl I noticed on that very afternoon wearing her grey sweater loosely. Her brown hair flitted about in the cool breeze swirling above our heads. I was moving my wheelchair nervously back and forth as we talked. The gentle clicks of the motors working somehow helped to calm me down like some giant metronome.

I gained an insight into her life as we exchanged 'war' stories of our different impairments. My problems with DMD and her problems walking and I think epilepsy but I'm not sure after all these years. It was good not to talk about hospitals or worry about germs and I hoped we took each other's mind off our problems. A wave of fiery emotion suddenly brewed deep in my heart and I plucked up a courage I never thought I had in me. In a determined carpe diem moment I looked into her sparkling brown eyes and asked, "… Do you want to go out with me? I … really … um … like you a lot …" The next moments seemed to drag on into eternity as she mulled over my request.

As I'd laid my heart on the line I immediately felt hot and uncomfortable whilst awaiting her reply. With a gleaming smile she confirmed that she liked me a lot too and tentatively agreed to be my girlfriend. I was very happy to have something I thought improbable, an actual girlfriend! I was excited beyond belief as I drove my wheelchair beside her, with a smile beginning to blossom across my face. We walked and drove towards the unit as we both had a free period. Often at the beginning of the autumn term it was very quiet with lots of free periods and thinking time between lessons. Suddenly she grasped my free hand as we proceeded down the white corridor and in turn this made me feel warm and fuzzy inside. Was this the love people talk of or was it just a teenage romance I wondered. It definitely felt like the former to me.

In order to protect the identity of my former romances I will refer to them as Miss A. Miss B. etc. I don't want them to be upset by what I may say. I obviously don't set out to upset any of them but I couldn't forgive myself for potentially trampling on people's feelings by revisiting awkward issues. Once inside the unit Miss A and I sat down together and looked at each other longingly. Just then Mrs Watkins entered the room from a coffee break she was having. She could see us holding each others hands and talking quietly whilst sitting next to the blue and white unit tables. She sat down beside us and as if by magic or some mysterious intuition quickly came to the conclusion that we were starting a relationship. Over the coming days she would regularly ask me about Miss A and when should she get her hat ready! We often giggled at that sentiment.

Soon it was time to go home on that beautiful late summer's afternoon. Before we each left to go to our separate ways for the evening I asked Miss A for her mobile phone number. I reluctantly released the grasp of my sweetheart's warm hand and boarded my taxi as she handed me the number. I was sad to be leaving her for the night but excited that we would meet up again the next day. On the way home I thought about what message to send to Miss A, for most of the afternoon we talked about music. I remember at the time the most popular song was by Kylie with her great sounding tune "Can't get you out of my head". I thought how apt as I couldn't get Miss A out of my head, so I imagined we'd continue our conversation on that topic. We would eventually text each other every night gaining yet more insight into each others minds; I loved her personality and sense of humour the most.

It wasn't long until my mother found out about the relationship. She had to pick me up from school one grey afternoon and while we waited for the taxi she met Miss A. We all talked to each other about various things like where Miss A lived. She lived in the opposite direction to us living near Cardiff, whereas I obviously lived in Abercynon. Miss A was down that day as either her leg or stomach were in pain, so she didn't say an awful lot to my mother. I didn't think she was expecting to meet one of my parents so early on but she handled it very well in my opinion. My mother said on the way home that she thought Miss A was a little gloomy or grumpy, she didn't sound very enthusiastic about her at all. I didn't think she was overly unhappy, it was just the way she was. I had no problems at all with her and she seemed so perfect and genuine to me. We were good sounding boards to each others frustrations and we didn't need to mention our impairments we just saw through that.

At the weekend we texted each other a lot more and if we got tired with that then we phoned and listened quietly to each others voices. I really liked listening to her soft voice floating through the receiver. I just loved talking about everything unrelated to DMD; there was no mention of germs, no mention of my ever increasing paralysis. Overall I was extremely happy as opposed to being so distressed and desperately ill just a few short weeks ago. We both wondered what was coming up for us over the next week, I told her how tough sixth form was going to be and she wondered what career I might like to go into. It was a question I had so much trouble answering as I had no idea and wondered what if any employer would take me on. On a pleasant note we ended the weekend full of excitement about meeting up in school the next morning. No Monday morning blues for us as these were truly happy times.

Unbeknownst to me that day was to be my last ever in St Cenydd School. I can remember that it was quite wet that Monday morning I only just managed to avoid the worst of the rain falling from the leaden skies. I stayed in the sixth form building most of the day keeping myself warm and dry. I sat with Miss A during our free periods and we talked about various things including our mobile phone cases which were interchangeable and in many different colours (I am a bit of a technological geek so I found this feature most appealing). It felt like a really slow day as I watched the students milling about in between their lessons. It was so enjoyable passing the time holding hands with Miss A; it was almost cosy on that damp day. If only there was a fireplace to warm our hearts by it would have just set the scene off perfectly.

My last enduring memory of sixth form life was an impromptu gig that one of my peers called Michael (who is extremely good on the guitar) set up. He was taking requests and thrashing out tunes that people were throwing at him. I was over awed by his talent as the songs definitely sounded like they should have, if not better than the real thing. His beautifully crafted and mellow sounding acoustic guitar was delightfully purring in his arms. I wished that I knew a proper guitar song to request but I just couldn't think of anything on the spot. By the time I thought of a possible song another student would jump in and ask Michael to play one of their favourite tunes. Despite this I was happy just to listen whilst continuing to hold hands with Miss A. There's nothing better than hearing live music in an intimate setting. At least I ended my school life on a high note with a great lasting memory.

Tuesday September the eleventh 2001 was momentous in many ways. I remember with incredulity watching the terrible attack on the twin towers in New York City. My mother thought the news broadcast was a film or even a documentary. I told her "No Mam, this is happening now!" it was totally surreal as that fateful day elapsed. The incredible grounding of every plane and the equally awful attack on the pentagon all pressed deeply on our minds. That day changed the world so much for everyone including me.

I was home on that stressful day as I felt unwell and again with a terrible fright I could feel some secretions building up. No amount of huffing or tapping my chest made me feel any better. I was very much hoping to avoid getting worse, I could just about manage to breathe sitting up in my wheelchair. As the evening approached I had to make an uncomfortable decision. Could I manage to last the night struggling to breathe and feeling generally unwell or did I have to visit the hospital. I agonised about this question for a good few hours I was so worried that the secretions starting to rattle in my lungs would turn catastrophic again. I also worried that if I went into hospital I would somehow be wasting the doctors' time. I came to a decision when my father said "So what are we going to do then Ian? …" In a sudden fight or flight moment I weighed up the options, I just knew I wouldn't last the night without medical intervention.

"We're going to have to go to the hospital ... because I think ... I won't last the night" I said in a shaky bravado stricken voice. Immediately we proceeded to my van which was parked across the street from our house. It was a cool early evening as I was raised into the van by my father. Again we took that same route which snaked its way down the dual carriageway towards the motorway and Llandough beyond. It was a very quiet journey toward the hospital as I was just trying to control my breathing. The fluid in my lungs became even thicker and again my weak cough came back to haunt me. The evening light was fast dimming as the forty minute ride came to an end.

We arrived again at the children's ward with its murals plastering the windows. I really wished there was an adolescent ward. Although I didn't care at that precise moment as I drove through the main doors in my Harrier wheelchair. This time the nurse's allowed me to stay in my wheelchair as I told them it was easier to breathe that way. I explained my breathing difficulties and the fluid mucus floating painfully in my throat. I can remember the physiotherapists being called out; they tried everything on me including guiding me through some coughing exercises and tapping my chest wall. These attempts were only compounding my problems as the secretions were getting heavier and heavier.

I was getting exhausted and more distressed by the minute. The nurses tried to make things easier by putting me in a bed but no matter what position they hoisted me into I could get no relief whatsoever. The physiotherapists came back to try again on my chest but this time they brought medical machinery with them. I had no idea what I was supposed to do but a small pipe was placed in my mouth and I was told to breathe in a mysterious cloudy gas. In the beginning this was helping me to breathe which made my chest feel a lot easier. This was short lived however as I kept asking for more and more of this helpful gas to soothe my lungs. By now the machine had reached at its maximum setting and was soon struggling to keep up.

I began to feel so tired and distressed as my breathing started to get worse overpowering the machine I was breathing on. "I need the *Nippy* ... ugh ... I'm so tired dad ... I just need the *Nippy*!" I whispered out in tears to my father. I kept repeating my request to use the Nippy ventilator. Eventually after seeing me struggle to breathe and as the physiotherapists machines failed, the nurses had no option but to send me up to intensive care. Once wheeled there in the hospital bed two specialist nurses attached the claustrophobic mask and headgear to my face. I was locked in again to the dependant world I thought I left behind back in May. However I just knew I would feel better once that cool streaming air was pumped into me.

The Nippy was eventually turned on and immediately I relaxed as the high pressure air squeezed in; I was literally eating the air down. I could finally close my eyes as the predictable breaths formed a rhythm that gently 'rocked' me off to sleep. The air was forcing the newly formed secretions down into the far reaches of my chest. It felt as if my lungs were a small caisson with the fluids pushed away under high pressure. Again I had IV drips inserted into my arm around the wrist area as my elbow contractures stopped the nurses accessing their usual area. An arterial line was also inserted into my right wrist to allow for easier blood taking. I was so tired and 'out of it' that I hardly noticed the nurses inserting the needles.

I had a stable night in intensive care as the ventilator supported my overworked muscles. Doctor Hebden came in around mid morning to discuss my case and check on my progress. The nurses managed to briefly take me off the *Nippy* so I could talk things over about my current condition. I explained the worrying secretions had come back and that I was unable to cough them away. Doctor Hebden felt that I ought to have the mini tracheotomy reinserted into my neck so the fluid secretions could be removed with suction. This time however I was much more awake and alert meaning I would be more aware during the procedure that doctor Hebden would carry out. He wanted to try inserting the mini tracheotomy without using a sedative, presumably because of the muscle relaxant effect it may have had upon me which can be dangerous for DMD patients.

I was prepared for the small operation/procedure by one friendly nurse who I got on with really well; she covered me in that green fabric you often see on those television medical programmes. Doctor Hebden carefully felt my neck searching for the exact and crucial spot the incision for a mini tracheotomy could be made. Next my neck was cleaned and slightly numbed to take the edge off things. He then brought over a small scalpel ready to make the incision in the spot he had earlier marked. I was told to keep my head still and not to talk while the cut was made into my neck.

I could feel the pressure applied to my neck when the first cuts were made but only felt a very small amount of pain, the numbing agent must have worked. I could however feel the warm blood flowing down the front of my neck and onto my chest and this was a most unpleasant experience. I found breathing to be most awkward as my head and neck were in an unnatural position. After what seemed an age of careful manoeuvring and cutting doctor Hebden had finally produced the stoma necessary for a mini tracheotomy to be inserted. I could feel the air escaping through my nose and the newly formed hole, which made breathing seem slightly harder as the air inside my lungs leaked away faster.

Next the actual mini tracheotomy tube was brought over. As I said earlier it is a curved tube about four inches long. The end that is on the outside of my neck looks like two blue "butterfly" wings with a cap sticking out in the middle. The inside tube is made of clear plastic with a numbered graduation pattern stamped on (this is commonly found on a syringe and some other measuring devices). When the mini tracheotomy is renewed or first inserted a device called an introducer is used. The introducer is a hollow tube or needle which fits inside the mini tracheotomy it is also longer and thinner than the mini tracheotomy and quite draconian in its appearance. A thin silvered wire is also used when the mini tracheotomy is first inserted or renewed.

The final stage to completing the procedure is as follows. The silvered wire is fed down the hole in my throat and the introducer with the mini tracheotomy attached is brought to the free end of the wire. Next the hollow introducer is covered in a water soluble lubricant and slid along the wire into my throat. It felt as if my whole windpipe was blocked but before I could think about that the introducer along with the silvered wire was quickly removed leaving the mini tracheotomy behind in my throat. Finally a tracheotomy tube holder is placed around my neck and fastened into place on the blue "butterfly" wings. Unfortunately a heck of a lot of blood had poured out of the new wound and I could see by doctor Hebden's face that he wasn't entirely happy with how the procedure went. Indeed he told me later that if I needed it done again he would not do it with me fully aware. I agreed even though I hoped I wouldn't need to experience this yet again.

Everything was much easier in terms of secretion removal after the insertion of my second mini tracheotomy. I felt immediately better and was able to tolerate the *Nippy* ventilator longer overnight. I improved so much that by the end of the week I was moved out of intensive care and back onto the children's ward. I was immensely happy to see my family once again; it was so hard being stuck on intensive care as visiting times were so short. My recovery was quite astonishing given how ill I was on September the eleventh. Eventually the doctors were considering the removal of the mini tracheotomy once again. I had mixed feelings about this suggestion as I was worried that the fluid secretions would immediately come back. On the other hand though I didn't want to have a hole in my neck, I was scared of drowning in the bath or getting the tube caught on something.

I stayed in the hospital for two weeks to give my chest a chance to recover enough to remove the trachy. I had finished a protective antibiotic course by the end of my stay. I had one of the best children's doctors in my opinion, called doctor Alfaham. I would make him laugh by the things I often said about the treatments he would suggest. One comical incident happened when he described a drug called Domperidone but I thought he said Don Perignon the Champagne! He was in fits of laughter and liked my expensive tastes, we all laughed at that. He was an amazing kindly doctor who was an expert with children and with me as an older teenager. I am grateful for his time and caring nature, his staff also did an excellent job taking care of my medical needs.

All too soon the trachy was removed and once again my neck could be cleaned by my mother. The dried red blood was quite hard to scrub off as it was firmly caked into my throat. Again the hole or stoma in my neck quickly receded and eventually no trace of it could be found. I had one last scare however on the day before I was due to leave. Again I could feel secretions building up in my lungs and I was getting increasingly worried and scared by this eventuality. Quickly a physiotherapist was called out to help me try and cough it up. He was a kind Irish man who helped me to calm down as panicking definitely wouldn't help. Next he used a nebuliser to thin out the secretions floating in my windpipe. Eventually with breathing exercises and some gentle coughs I managed to clear my chest and finally breathe easier.

Shortly after my chest was cleared we left the hospital travelling in my van back to our house in Abercynon. I was given a *Nippy* ventilator to take home just incase I had another turn for the worse to put my mind at ease. It was around this time that I officially left school because of the dangers of other potentially ill people making me unwell yet again. I was relieved to be leaving the stress behind and it was a huge weight off my shoulders. When the stress was piled on me I would worry to a point nearing lunacy. This in turn would leave me at a low ebb and crucially susceptible to even the most minor cold. I worried about my future prospects but I really was having a battering over the course of 2001. My disease really had taken a huge turn for the worse and I had to grow up quickly. There was no more naivety about my illness I definitely took it a lot more seriously.

I missed one person the most during my stay in hospital. I quickly texted Miss A as soon as I got home from my ordeal and it was good to finally explain what happened. I hadn't been able to use my phone during my stay because of hospital policy surrounding mobile phones. Miss A had missed me quite a lot or so it seemed at the time until I got a rather curious message. "When are you coming back to school?" she texted me one dark grey afternoon, I found this most difficult to answer. I wrestled myself to find the words to message back with; I thought she knew the answer to that question already. I struggled to explain that I was just too ill to return to school and the stress of sixth form was doing me no good. She answered that with a short and sweet "Ok" and I thought that was that and we were 'cool'. I hoped she still loved me and that I didn't need to be in school for things to still work out.

Things became strained after that conversation by text message. Miss A seemed to message and telephone far more infrequently. I was always asking if anything was wrong and had I said something to upset her. I would get snappy answers saying nothing had changed and not to be silly. Indeed things seemed to stabilise slightly after my initial concerns. In due course we began texting regularly as if the last few weeks were a dream until one cold autumn night. I got a most nonchalant text message simply stating that our relationship was over. I got the usual "it's not you, it's me" statement that you read about in magazines. I was stunned by this straightforward and direct message and was getting quite upset inside. I could only manage a "well, if you're sure" message after that bombshell. I also pleaded with her "are you sure we can't work this out?" "No" was the answer and Miss A confirmed that our relationship was indeed over. I was sat in my lounge in a numbed cruel silence I could hardly believe what had just happened.

She never texted me again after that impersonal dumping and I felt totally lost and confused. I didn't know how to feel, what had I done to deserve this. I cried a little as I rose up in my lift to my bedroom; I managed to compose myself before my mother saw me. I didn't want anybody to see how upset I was and I decided as my mother hoisted me into bed that I would just forget about it. That was totally easier said than done but I knew being upset and negative could only make me ill again. It was tough but a few days later I managed to get out of the depths of sadness and climb the heights of positivity that galvanises my life. In hindsight I suppose not many teenagers could manage a long distance relationship (even though it's less than fifteen miles) but I didn't know exactly what was going on in Miss A's life at that time. However it still hurt to be dumped via a text I don't know to this day why she couldn't have just rung me.

In cold way I had to forget about her and concentrate on myself. I was so determined not to get ill and wished so hard to be like other teenagers. Accepting the seriousness of my condition was very hard but I managed to take comfort in the things I could still do, namely playing my *Playstation 2*. I could block out the entire world sitting in my chair in the bedroom. It kept me sane and I could live out any fantasy I wanted from football supremo to boxing world champion. It really did make me happy I often extolled the pleasures of each individual game to my father most evenings. I would get so enthusiastic about the adventures of my day. I look back on those carefree afternoons with mixed feelings, I'm thrilled I was happy but a small part of me felt I should be moving on at least trying to get a career.

One Sunday morning in November I was sitting in my bed challenging my cousin to a game of football on the *Playstation 2*. We were having a fantastic fun time blasting shots from way out and laughing at our awful goalkeepers. It proceeded smoothly like this for about two hours until suddenly and unexpectedly I took a turn for the worse. I looked down to press a button on the game control when out of nowhere a coughing fit beset me. I was scared at that moment because my breathing immediately became difficult. My cousin was worried when he heard the awful noise emanating from my chest. He quickly ran to fetch my mother from the downstairs living room, calling out "Aunty Sue!!" as he ran.

She came rushing up the stairs to see if I was alright. I could immediately see that she was worried by the tone of her strained voice. "Mam, Its hurting my chest … I can't breathe!" I wailed out nervously. "Well let's put you in your chair, sitting awkwardly in that bed isn't helping you!" she strained. Once back in my chair she guided me through some huffing exercises while she began tapping my back. She would tap various spots on the back and front of my chest using 'cupped' hands in the hopes of moving some muck; we were taught this by the hospital physiotherapists. Eventually the noise on my chest seemed to quieten and indeed I began to feel a little better.

By the evening I noticed my breathing was becoming very difficult again. I was gasping and beginning to feel like I did in September. I wondered why this kept happening to me, I felt really low and stressed. I had to contemplate yet again whether or not to go to hospital. It was getting infuriatingly annoying getting ill every few weeks. It was tiring and extremely frightening always worrying about my breathing, one wrong move and my chest could erupt like it just had. However I made the decision to stay at home and try out the *Nippy* ventilator that had been left with us. I was going to see how I felt overnight and then check myself the next day.

"I want to try the nippy tonight Mam" I said in my nervous valley's accent. Eventually after a few nervous comments my mother agreed to try me on the ventilator. She managed to put the mask on whilst trying to avoid over tightening it. She attached the tube to the front of the mask and switched the machine on. At first nothing happened until a loud ear splitting screech started blaring. My mother had accidently left it unplugged so she frantically reinserted it and the deafening noise ceased. I'm sure the whole street heard it that late autumn evening. The familiar cool pressurised air started forcing its way into my lungs with its monotonous rhythm. "Ah!" I said as my lungs began inflating and then quickly deflating; I often start my night with the same gasp of relief even now.

The next day I felt terrible as I came off the ventilator. My lungs felt quite odd indeed I couldn't hear any noise but I felt as if I was breathing through tar. My nose was blocked and my throat felt dry and coarse. Every now and then when I needed it my mother would wipe my nose, sickly green mucus was left behind in the tissue. Suddenly with a cold realisation I knew I was ill. To be on the safe side I had to go back to the hospital yet again. I couldn't risk secretions building up to levels where I could potentially choke. Again my father would have to immediately drive me down to Llandough hospital.

We made the usual trip down the dual carriageway onto the motorway and the hospital beyond. This time we were prepared for the long haul by bringing my own mobile hoist, my own *Nippy* ventilator and a travel bag. In the bag were some spare clothes, a roll of kitchen towel (as I was dribbling quite profusely), all of my prescriptions and pumps. I felt quite low as we belted along the motorways watching the golden orange autumn trees fly by. The low annoying sun burned in my eyes which made them tear over. I asked my mother for a hug as we neared the hospital, I was really weary of going back there; I could almost smell that horrible disinfectant.

My white van shining like a beacon passed through Llandough's main entrance. It wasn't long until I wearily drove my chair onto the children's ward into one of their cubicles prepared nearby. The staff knew I was coming because my father had rung ahead earlier to warn of my immanent arrival. Again I was hoisted onto a bed this time using my comfortable hoist and sling. Next many questions were asked about my condition; it seemed that the nurses never remembered anything about DMD. I just wanted to be well and I often said "Do whatever it takes to make me feel better". I was taken down to x-ray to see what was stuck in my lungs; unsurprisingly the radiologist confirmed I had lots of fluid down there.

Over the next few hours I was given plenty of strong antibiotics intravenously. I must have been a guinea pig to about half a dozen student doctors; they had a great deal of difficulty inserting needles into both of my wrists. On one occasion my right ankle was used as a potential IV site; it absolutely hurt like hell. I'm sure I could feel it slide against my bone, thank goodness they removed that one! By the evening doctor Hebden came around to see why I was in the hospital yet again. I explained my current predicament of how every few weeks secretions were returning to my chest with no way of me shifting them. I also divulged how tired and worn down I was as my breathing weighed very heavily on my mind.

Taking all of these considerations into hand doctor Hebden offered me a solution out of my secretion problems. He suggested that I have a mini tracheotomy permanently fitted into my neck. This prompted a barrage of questions from us; I specifically asked "Will it make me more prone to infections?" To which doctor Hebden replied "There is a risk whenever the cap is opened as you're avoiding the body's airway defence system". However he thought the benefits of clearing my airways certainly outweighed the risks posed by infection as long as we used the correct clean procedure. That was enough to convince me to go ahead with the procedure; I wanted to stop this endless procession of hospital visits.

My mother was initially apprehensive as she would presumably have to suck my chest out the most being my main carer and all. The physiotherapists especially a beautiful blonde lady called Ann put her mind at rest. She reassured my mother about the technique which could be easily learnt. After their initial concerns my parents were keen for me to have the mini tracheotomy procedure; they could see I was struggling and generally distressed by the constant bouts of illness. We further discussed the implications of my proposed permanent mini tracheotomy with doctor Hebden. This brought up the fact that the actual plastic tracheotomy device had to be changed monthly. I wasn't looking forward to this but like I had said earlier I'd do whatever it takes.

The next day I was wheeled up to intensive care on the cold steel hospital bed. It was a bright sunny day with shafts of golden light shining through the blinds. I was confronted by doctor Hebden and an anaesthetist who happened to be from Aberdare which was only a few miles from my house. Standing next to the anaesthetist was a large machine with two large dials and a pipe sticking out the front. It was explained to me that during this procedure I would be given gas and air (I'm not sure if that is correct term for what I was given). My bed was moved to the left of this machine and again I was prepared for the procedure with the same green fabric that was used just a few weeks prior.

My neck was cleaned while I nervously chatted to the staff surrounding the bed. A few swift moments later doctor Hebden was ready to begin. The machine's pipe was brought over with a full face mask dangling on the end of it. The anaesthetist put the mask over my face and I could smell the strange colourless gas pumping out of the pipe. I closed my eyes thinking that I was supposed to do this but I was quickly admonished by the anaesthetist who said "No, Please keep your eyes open. Thanks mate". I quickly opened them and looked at one particular ceiling tile. As I was doing this I fell into a curious trance where I could feel nothing, see nothing apart from the tile and I couldn't hear a thing. Moments later and as if Sigmund Freud had snapped his fingers I was self aware again.

"Are you done, is it in?" I inquired of the doctors. I listened in mild confusion as I was told that everything went successfully. I was in complete surprise as it only seemed I was in a trance for one or two seconds. I tilted my head down and could just feel the scratchy cap of the mini tracheotomy rasping at my chin. I felt really tired after the small procedure and soon the nurses put my *Nippy* mask back on so I could have a rest. They also checked my oxygen saturations and would often clear my chest through the newly inserted mini tracheotomy. I remained stable through the night as the ventilator whirred away. The antibiotics coursing through my veins were making me feel so much better; most of my cold symptoms had disappeared completely.

By the third day on intensive care I was again told that I was "too well to be in ICU". Quickly my bed was wheeled back down to the children's ward where again I was reunited with my parents. I asked my mother for a hug (I have to ask because I am unable to move my arms) I was really happy to get out of intensive care. I had been there three times that year alone, thankfully I have never gone back but as I now know anything could happen. It is always worrying to think that one single infection could potentially and quickly turn into something horrid which could put me right back in intensive care. I try as hard as I can to bury the worry into the back of mind and adopt a sort of bravado approach of "I can avoid this!" Positive determination helps me a lot these days, I want to avoid negativity or I'll get depressed and probably ill. Some days I have to put that smile on my face or I just couldn't go on.

I would have gone home soon after my return to the ward had it not been for a terrible bout of constipation. I know this isn't the most pleasant of things to discuss but it can happen quite a lot with some Duchenne's patients. The powerful antibiotics had a very strong binding effect and combined with the propensity of DMD to cause problems in this particular area I indeed got constipated. It is the single most painful thing that I suffer with amongst all the problems I face. It was agonising sitting in my chair as my body tried to move the blockage, but when I try to 'go', I push and push and push to no avail only wearing myself out more. Whenever I coughed pain would reverberate throughout my whole body. On one particular occasion I burst into tears in front of a physio who was working on my chest. Another problem is that I can't urinate without wanting to 'do' the other thing so my bladder feels constantly and painfully full. All of this caused me to become extremely frustrated and in particular nasty to everyone, I couldn't help it and I suppose it's understandable given the pain I was in.

The nurses tried various medications to help me pass the excruciating blockage; including magnesium salts, Senna (a natural remedy), Lactulose (a sort of oil that is supposed to soften stools) and other laxatives. Nothing seemed to work and all the solutions made me feel sick. This in turn put me right off food which only compounded my problems further. As I was just about to give up all hope the nurses tried the last weapon in their arsenal. I was going to have the pleasure of an enema! I didn't really care what they did as long as they made me feel better. I couldn't take this pain anymore so the nurses had to do something.

At around five in the afternoon a nurse called Helen brought in the equipment. I was rolled on to my stomach which made my breathing so difficult and uncomfortable. I couldn't really see anything but I sure as heck felt it as the enema delivery system was thrust into position. I screamed out in agony and I'm sure I woke people up in the next room. I thought I was going to quickly pass out but I just managed to control myself before the liquid was pumped in. The pain dropped down many notches as the solution entered my body. An excruciating fifteen minutes passed by until Helen removed the delivery system. I was quickly rolled onto my back gulping down mouthfuls of air in the process. I didn't feel any different except that my stomach felt like the size of a beach ball.

I had a pretty uneventful night sleeping in the warm hospital room up until around three as I literally exploded in the bed; it was an amazing relief to be finally rid of the blockage that had made my life a living hell. In a meek and shaky voice I said "Mam I think I had an accident!" we always laugh about this moment as my face was a picture. Quickly and quietly my mother hoisted me up into the air and cleaned everything she also took the dirty sheets to the hospital sluice. It was such a powerful reaction that my sling got covered in the process so my mother took it off and the nurses tried to clean it. Luckily there was a washing machine on the ward and not long after we had a freshly washed and warm sling given back to us.

Five weeks after I had gone into the hospital I was finally discharged. Before we left my mother was taught the clean technique for suctioning out my chest. Basically you use one 'clean' hand that is in a sterile glove to feed the suction tube down the trachy (my abbreviated term for the mini tracheotomy). Whilst the other 'dirty' hand does everything else including opening the catheter sheaf a small amount and attaching the actual tube onto the suction machine. Also the 'dirty' hand covers a small connector that activates the suction machine which in turn sucks the mucus out of my lungs. The tube is slowly pulled out whilst I'm being suctioned and when the catheter is removed the whole process starts afresh. It didn't take my mother too long to learn the technique; I learnt the theory so that I could teach others to do it in emergencies.

The very last person we met before departing was the respiratory nurse who would be changing my trachy every month. She is a lovely tall lady with dark hair called Paula who still visits me to change the trachy every now and then as part of a bigger team. I first met her when she came to the hospital room I was staying in to run through the instructions of the *Nippy* ventilator. At first we didn't know what to make of her as she whirled through the ventilator directions but after awhile we came to respect her and I truly think she's a wonderful person. Paula really seems to understand what caring for a person entails. I've experienced a lot of nurses who see caring as job; like a stack 'em, pack 'em and rack 'em system rather than a vocation of true care that Paula definitely understood.

Finally I could board my van and leave the children's ward behind for good (it was closing in the coming year to be replaced by a Cystic Fibrosis ward). I was very happy to be going home as the New Year was fast approaching. I had a new hope that I wouldn't always be coming into hospital to stay and that my new trachy would allow me far more freedom. This was the beginning of yet another change in my life it was now going to be full of ventilators and suction machines and the worry of possibly getting ill. At least now I had a bit of reassurance from the new trachy and I hoped happier times were ahead.

# Age Eighteen

The weeks and months following my discharge and leading up to my eighteenth birthday were quite difficult for my mother and me. We were fine with the clean procedure of suctioning but crucially I was struggling to know when to halt the process. Every time I thought my chest was clear of fluid and told my mother to remove the catheter, "Right, I'm done Mam" I would say but two or three minutes later I could hear and feel secretions again. This meant I had to redo suction much to my mothers' annoyance. After many stressful days I was finally learning my body's telltale signs and signals, when I said my chest was clear eight times out of ten it was. Tensions dropped noticeably and I settled into a pattern of one or two 'suctions' a week.

The only unfortunate issue concerned the gloves we used for the procedure. I was told that the health authority withdrew the single use *Dispos-A-Glove* brand we were used too; replacing them with a more expensive latex type. I wasn't willing to change what my mother and I had been taught to use back in 2001. The only option left for me was to buy them off a healthcare company I found on the internet, we pay around £100 for one thousand gloves or ten boxes every few weeks. On the rest of the supply front my local district nurses still provide the suction catheters for me to use; produced by *Pennine healthcare*. I use size ten catheters with black connection sockets and they have smooth ends (as opposed to ends with a small bubble on which are not mini tracheotomy compatible).

In my new steady pattern I could concentrate on the other things that mattered in my life namely family and a small amount of study. Sian had moved away to study textiles at the University of Wolverhampton where she would stay for approximately three years. She would regularly visit our home so she didn't miss us too much. Emma had returned to Wales to teach in a local 'special' school after teaching in Essex up until I was ill. She felt she was too far away if anything happened to me again. My sisters are very caring and protective towards me, after a difficult 2001 we were all a little 'closer' to one another.

My father was working his way up through the ranks at Cardiff University where he would eventually get his 'chair' and become a professor. My mother was doing an excellent job caring for me but was rarely getting a break. Luckily we received the service of an organisation of carers called *Crossroads* who in their remit 'care for carers'. Once a fortnight two kind carers would come in to sit with me while my parents went out for a few hours. They would either go to the cinema or to the Bingo in a nearby town, while at home I would talk and play games with the regular carers I had. The two carers were taught how to perform suction by a local physiotherapist so I didn't have to worry about that aspect of my care. Also a different carer who took me out every weekend was taught the technique, but sadly he couldn't try the procedure out because my local Social Services cut the facility and I lost my weekly excursions once and for all.

I had just finished studying with a tutor who guided me through the rest of my A/S level in Business Studies. I found it difficult to study as my concentration levels were really low and I had to switch examination boards from the *WJEC* (a Welsh exam board) to *AQA*. It had been a very tough year so I really didn't think there was any career out there for me even after the examination. I know many people will think that's a defeatist attitude to have but I had to face up to reality of my illness and condition. I was however interested in Business studies so I was determined to at least finish one course while I still could. I received my results just before my birthday attaining a D grade; my tutor told me I was one or two marks away from a C grade. I was glad that I had indeed what it takes to get a grade that wasn't equivalent to my disastrous U in Chemistry. I was slightly disappointed that I hadn't achieved a C but I could live with that.

July the fourteenth 2002 quickly arrived and I can remember how glorious a day it was. There wasn't a cloud in the bright cerulean sky and a hot sun shone strongly down upon my back garden. My father had organised a barbeque which most of my family attended including my uncle Alan, my cousins Sean and Sarah, my sisters Emma and Sian along with their boyfriends. It was great to see everyone there celebrating my ascension to adulthood. We partied well into the night playing many games and I experimented with my first proper pint of lager. The smell of dew and barbequed meat filled the air that night. The only bad part about me drinking was the fact I never shut-up! I talked for hours upon hours, laughing and giggling at the most inane things until my jaw began to ache from the effort.

I got some brilliant presents from my parents and family but I was just happy to see them; their presence was enough for me. However the best present I got came from my sister Sian. She bought me a Manchester United football shirt framed in a black and white surround. It has my first name in bold white letters with a large number 18 below it. The black frame complemented the striking red shirt really well. It still hangs on my bedroom wall now; it always makes me smile seeing it twinkling away in the corner every night. My eighteenth birthday was definitely one of the best birthday's I'd ever had and I was so happy Sian had got me a gift that I truly appreciated.

As mentioned in the last chapter my mini tracheotomy has to be changed every four to six weeks. Initially we went back to Llandough every month so that doctor Hebden (a tall, friendly, plaid shirted intensive care doctor) could perform the renewal process. To recap the process, a silvered wire is fed down my 'old' tracheotomy tube until it stimulates a cough. Next the 'old' tube is slowly pulled out along the wire (the wire stays in place). Next the combined draconian needle-like introducer tube and new mini tracheotomy (pre-lubricated) are brought over to the wire and fed down my throat. By now I'm coughing profusely and my eyes are watering as a reflex nerve in my trachea has become over stimulated. The introducer and wire are removed leaving the tracheotomy tube behind. Lastly a tube holder is strapped on to the blue 'butterfly' wings protruding either side of the main cap. After the process I need immediate suction to clear the excess fluid that my weak cough manages to dislodge and this always feels highly uncomfortable.

I'm often asked what suction feels like which I find desperately hard to convey but here goes. Imagine drowning and the liquid water (in the case of a pool, mucus in my case) sloshing about inside your windpipe, your body will try to cough it out and get you breathing again (I'm assuming you've been rescued from the water and battling to breathe). I get the exact same feeling and if my chest isn't sucked out the mucus builds up and can block my airway all together. When the suction catheter is fed down it feels like another kind of blockage but it doesn't generally hurt. When suction is engaged I get a certain amount of relief as the secretions are removed it's as if someone turned my air back on again. There are times where I can get pain for instance if the mini tracheotomy moves while a catheter is being fed down. Another worrying thing that has happened is if the suction catheter hits my trachea 'wall' it can suck out tissue and blood, it's frightening and often very painful when that takes place; but it happens very rarely. Sadly there's no way to know when that could happen next but as long as the catheter is fed down carefully, which it generally is, usually no trauma occurs.

After two or three changes Paula the senior respiratory nurse was taught the procedure and this meant that monthly changes could now take place in my home. This allows me not to have constant exposure to any bugs that are potentially lurking in the hospital. Also it saved my father having to book time off work every month to drive me to Llandough. At the start of these home changes I felt very apprehensive as I wasn't sure it would work. Generally Paula did a fantastic job considering she had just learnt the procedure. Initially it was quite difficult pushing the new mini tracheotomy's down the hole because of over granulation surrounding the stoma (excess skin) caused by my body as a means of rejection. It has since been controlled by a cream which effectively 'kills' it off.

On the very rare occasion a new tracheotomy could not be fitted I would have to be rushed down to Llandough by my father (he had to be called from work) so doctor Hebden could successfully re-install it. One particular moment shines brightly in my memory. Paula was teaching a nurse from a local hospital called Jon (a tall, dark haired bespectacled man) to install my latest tracheotomy. Unfortunately whilst trying to slide it down the silver wire, Jon accidently tried to put the mini tracheotomy in upside down! After many a confused moment he had to give up on the procedure as there was no way it could be fitted the wrong way up. Jon got very concerned and slightly panicky even suggesting an ambulance be called out.

Calmly and efficiently Paula and my mother took over, firstly gauze was placed on my neck protecting the stoma, my mother rang my father so that he could come home to take us back to Llandough. My father arrived around thirty or so minutes later in his red *Ford* car.

Next I would meet him round the back of the house and together we would proceed to our white *VW* van parked outside near the back door. I rode the lift up to the van's side door and reversed into position in the middle of the vehicle. My parents and I set off towards the hospital with Paula following behind in her car. Meanwhile Jon who had failed in his attempt to insert the mini tracheotomy made his way back to his workplace at the local hospital. He later pointed us in the direction of the previously mentioned cream for the over granulation surrounding my stoma and I'm very grateful for that.

After a whirlwind drive we arrived at Llandough hospital some forty minutes later, Paula was amazed by how fast my father got us there as we made excellent time. During the journey my index finger was plugged into an oxygen saturation monitor. As we proceeded down the various roads I saw my oxygen levels drop from ninety six percent down to a much lower eighty four percent (anything over ninety being normal). The monitor was sounding an alarm as my levels continued drop. My chest was noisy and beginning to fill with fluid, I tried to remain calm and not worry by using some exasperated humour. "Oh shut up you silly bloody thing! I know its 84!" I jokingly shouted at the monitor. Making up jokes and other amusements took mind my off the issue and helped the journey fly by.

In no time at all I was driving my wheelchair into intensive care to meet up with doctor Hebden. Quickly and without a great deal of fuss he inserted a fresh plastic mini tracheotomy into the hole halfway up my throat. Finally and with a huge amount of relief my mother suctioned away the excess and potentially dangerous secretions rattling in my windpipe. The white mucus would literally 'shoot' up the suction tubing with a gurgling sound that only signalled to me pure relief. Moments later with a clear chest I was laughing and joking with my parents, doctor Hebden and Paula. Luckily after this failed tracheotomy change no further accidents occurred as Paula really learnt the renewal process off to a tee, so much so she has successfully trained several other respiratory nurses who often change my tracheotomy now.

As I settled into the monthly pattern of mini tracheotomy changes and general recuperation I developed a drastically different daily routine. I had to sleep throughout the night on the *Nippy* ventilator so I would awake locked behind the confining and often painful mask. Having my face enclosed in a mask presented an unforeseen problem, due to my voice being quite weak it was impossible for me to call my mother to help me out of bed. We solved this problem by purchasing a doorbell with a wireless button press unit. Unfortunately this was only a temporary measure as my hands became weaker and weaker meaning I could no longer press the chunky doorbell button. I now have an environmental control with a small light touch button that operates my bed, a phone and crucially a pager I can alert my mother with.

Once awake at around eleven (as opposed to the quarter past seven early school day starts I left behind a couple years prior) I would alert my mother by pressing the button nestling in my right hand. Shortly after my mother would climb the stairs, slide the door open and enter my room. She would open my curtains letting in tons of blazing sunshine or usually (as I live in Wales) gallons of rain and grey cloud would greet me. Next she took my mask off extremely carefully avoiding any sudden movements which could accidently hurt my nose. The skin on the bridge of my nose had broken down badly due to the poorly fitting mask I was given, it often bled quite a lot. Luckily a few years later I received a much better mask which cured that problem and the bridge of my nose recovered as best as it could but unfortunately I still have a scar there.

It would take me two or three minutes to get accustomed to my surroundings and fully wake up. Next my mother would rest kitchen towel on my stomach; this was due to me needing to 'spit' or dribble away excess mucus that would get clogged down the back of throat. The *Nippy* ventilator has a tendency to dry my mouth out forcing some mucus to collect in that area so I need to clear it every morning. Once that unpleasant business was complete it was time for me to be hoisted into my wheelchair. My mother hooks the grey sling surrounding my body onto the metal crossbar hanging from the hoist and I'm raised up into the air. My arms are carefully positioned on my legs so that my shoulders won't hurt. Next I'm moved over my wheelchair by the touch of the button and carefully lowered in.

Thus my day would begin with me sitting in the wheelchair in my blue walled bedroom. I would do the same thing day in day out and that was to play on my *Playstation 2* whilst my television twinkled away in the background. I suppose many people would be thinking how 'cool' it was to play games everyday, but I wasn't doing this with my feet up eating junk food. No it was either play on my games or do absolutely nothing letting my brain vegetate in front of the mind numbing television. I did often wonder was there more I could be doing but I had to remember how badly my body dealt with stress. I just couldn't face getting ill all over again.

While I played games up in my room my mother made me breakfast. Back then I usually ate spaghetti hoops on toast. My mother had to feed me because I am unable to move my arms off my wheelchair table. She would slowly put the food in my mouth and after an age chewing frantically I would just manage to swallow it down. I always drink *Pepsi Max* with meals via a straw; my father made me a block of wood for my drinks to be rested on which brought it nearer my mouth. I would talk about any news or interesting dreams in between mouthfuls of tasty food. If I wasn't in a particularly talkative mood I would just concentrate on my favourite football game (*Pro Evolution Soccer*). I took it quite seriously setting targets for myself and generally keeping my mind occupied.

The afternoon brought with it a light lunch of tuna sandwiches and again my mother would have to feed me. I had no problem accepting this part of my life; I knew I couldn't feed myself so it was either that or go hungry. As I've said in previous chapters I loved my mothers' sandwiches which filled me up just right. After I'd finished my sandwiches I would settle in for an afternoon of games and some interesting television documentaries. *Sky TV* was recently installed so I didn't have to watch the same daytime programming which threatened to numb my young mind. My favourite afternoon documentary was 'Local Heroes' presented by Adam Hart Davis a medium built bespectacled man with gradually greying hair. He would rove around the nation on his fluorescent bicycle describing various people who in their lives contributed greatly in the fields of science and technology. I learnt more about science from the likes of Davis and his ilk than I did in school; I could learn about new subjects at my own pace and without pressure.

At around five thirty in the afternoon I would finish up watching my science documentaries. I would get so bored and frustrated playing football by then and my hands would stiffen up a lot. I would call my mother (later paging her using the previously mentioned environmental control) and she would help me get into the lift. She would need to move my arm over to the wheelchair controls and turn my *Playstation 2* off. I would then drive reversing toward my old servant of a lift; my mother would open its doors and I'd drive in. Sixty seconds later I would arrive downstairs in the extension. Driving past the bathroom, through the kitchen and into the lounge I'd find my favourite spot to park. I would usually park by the first armchair I came across, it points toward a large television sitting in the far corner.

Once safely ensconced in my position I would wait for my father to return home. When he came in I would greet him with the same "Alright Dad?" every night.

He would say "Alright E how was your day?" E is what everyone in my family shortens my name too. We would then exchange stories about our day before dinner; I would wax lyrical about my football game endeavours and would list all my days' achievements. We would sometimes talk about science and his current topic which is waste management. I would carry on talking but often due to a hard days work he would slowly fall asleep watching television. All the while my mother busily prepared our evening meal.

I pretty much ate the same dinner every night that consisted of battered cod and *Birdseye* potato fritters. It was the only thing I could chew at the time so my parents had to make sure there was a ready supply. Every weekend my father made a trip to the supermarket on what was affectionately known as "the fritter run". He would trawl the aisles looking for the four or five packets I needed to make sure I had dinner each night. Again my mother would feed me while I supped on a chilled *Pepsi Max* between mouthfuls. After half an hour eating I would be finished and feeling quite full. I would then watch television from seven onwards; either a film or the consumer affairs programmes on most evenings.

The evening would drag on into the night but my father would go up to bed at around ten thirty, leaving me and my mother watching the television. Often my mother would knit making quaint little jackets for my fathers' colleagues' newborn babies and later her future grandchildren (my future nephew and niece). She has quite a talent for making the tiny little outfits in various colours ranging from white to pink to blue. I'm always amazed by the speed at which she churns out the patterns with that familiar clink of the needles. She used patterns out of her old seventies knitting books which were crumpled and browned by their near constant use. Also I would make my daily visit to the toilet at around this time, I spent quite a long time trying to force myself to go whilst hanging over the toilet in my hoist. I've always had difficulty going ever since I became a full time wheelchair user and also the way in which DMD attacks every muscle must have something to do with it.

A few hours later the clock would tick past midnight and I'd be starting to feel weary. Ever since I was ill I've felt the need to always see the next day in. I have a subconscious irrational worry about dying before a new day starts, I can't really pinpoint why this happens but I feel more comfortable watching the clock signal a new day. Usually my mother would lay down on our settee waiting for me to alert her as to when I was eventually ready to sleep. I now have a laptop computer to keep me occupied instead of just watching the late night documentaries provided on *Sky TV*.

After an hour or so I would be finally ready to call time on my day. Once the television (later the laptop) was switched off my mother would move my hand over to the wheelchair control and turn the chair on. I usually make my way to the bathroom where I sometimes cleaned my teeth (now I use mouthwash every night). My mother would move the electric brush over the section of teeth I told her to clean and two minutes later it would be all over. I spat out the excess toothpaste into a small plastic bowl filled with water as I could no longer reach the sink. Finally and before it was time to ride my lift back to the top floor of our house I would take my asthma pump and have a small gulp of soft drink.

Again the journey up in the lift was another sixty second affair filled with vibrations and strange clunking noises. Once upstairs I would nudge the outer door with my footplate and drive into my pleasantly warm bedroom meeting up with my mother. I usually get hoisted into bed next briefly stopping so my mother could scratch various parts of my legs that felt itchy as there was no way I could do it. Once I was comfortably in bed ensconced under my duvet I would talk over things that happened throughout my day. While my mother and I talked she would prepare my mask ready for my nightly sleep on the *Nippy* Ventilator. Eventually after careful jostling my mask would be securely fastened onto my face and the air initiated, I would slowly drift into a deep sleep whilst clutching the switch in my right hand. This was my usual daily routine for a few years.

A month or two into 2003 Sian visited home from university with her then current boyfriend, a medium built guy with black hair and a distinctive face. I never really got on well with the guy, he seemed quite full of himself and when we talked we would descend into a petty argument about sport. I mostly tried to ignore him hoping he was more mature with Sian (he wasn't as it turned out). In the evenings he would start drinking lager from small green bottles; this in turn would make him irritable and argumentative. I made sure that there was something interesting to watch on television hoping we could talk about that instead of venting about sport.

I love sport but I certainly didn't want to argue about it every night he was there.

However during one late afternoon he started a discussion that I really didn't anticipate. Whilst I was playing a driving game on the *Playstation 2* he came into my room and sat on my bed. He and Sian had recently got back from an afternoon in Cardiff. His conversation started off cordially enough with the usual query about my computer games and inevitably sport. Quickly he segued on to the topic of 'responsibility', he went on to ask me "How are you going to repay your parents for all the hard work and sacrifices they have made for you?" At the time I pretty much ignored his comment with a "Yeah, I suppose I'll find a way" I knew it was highly improbable that I'd get a job because I was and still am ill.

In the coming days I increasingly began to think about his words; I could hear the discussion replaying in my mind over and over again. I used to think irrationally that my father was expecting me to actually get a job and a degree. It made me feel nervous and my stomach would churn away until I focussed my mind on the latest computer game I happened to own. Often before bed I would ask my mother if more was expected of me but she always said "you're doing just fine as you are". It still didn't stop me genuinely feeling like I was letting people down by my failure to earn a living.

It was my father who came to the rescue which snapped me out of the hopelessness I felt. He must have seen I was worried by the constant concerned look I had plastered on my face. One non eventful evening my father came into my room passed the sliding door and sat in the same place that Sian's boyfriend had a few days earlier. I asked straightaway was there something I should be doing in terms of looking for a possible job or more education. In a touching gesture my father washed away all my fears in an instant. "I'm happy as long as you're happy son" he said, also he went on to say that if all I could do was play on my *Playstation 2* that would be fine. I am ill after all (even though I dislike saying I'm ill, it's counterintuitive to how I think but my body doesn't lie). Sian's now ex-boyfriend (they split acrimoniously) was completely wrong.

That brief period of uncertainty had made me wonder was there more to come for my life; looking up at the years ahead of me I just couldn't see me sat in front of a games machine. For the time being I was content and quite happy to continue on as before. Sian's ex's words had only strengthened our family bond not eroded it; there was no pressure on me in terms of getting a job. There were plenty of other problems associated with my disease that I and my family had to contend with. It was something that a stranger who knew nothing of the devastating effects of DMD could not understand.

As the months proceeded spring had sprung and the first flowers of the year began to grasp at the sunlight. For me I was facing a few more worrying weeks as I had my first really bad cold since coming home from hospital just a short year or so earlier. It was frightening as once again my lungs would fill with thick mucus and my ineffective cough would only aggravate the situation further. This time however I had a weapon to fight the secretions and that was my suction machine (at the time a *Laerdal Suction Unit*) which could suck away the infected mucus. The only major problem was that I needed suctioning far more often as much as twenty to thirty times a day; this was due to the continual deterioration common in DMD. Unfortunately this put a lot of strain upon my mother.

The usual procedure at the time whenever I got ill was to yet again proceed back to Llandough hospital. Once there I got assessed by either my consultant Dr. Gelder (a dark haired, slightly tall man who reminded me of Lars Tharp from the *Antiques Roadshow* he's left Llandough lately however) or by a doctor on site. Then I am given strong antibiotics to help me fight off the infection as my immune system is impaired quite a lot. They are not prepared to admit me into hospital as my chances of getting another worse infection are greatly increased. Generally I was told to go home, drink lots more fluids also take some soluble paracetamol and continue on my course of antibiotics. I was advised to go on my ventilator more if I became extremely tired and struggled to breathe which always tends to happen.

Back home I would begin the often painful recovery period that could last up to two months. I remember one medium built blonde respiratory nurse called Angela; telling me that in some cases it can take up to three months to fully recover from a chest infection. It's a daunting prospect which makes me dread ever getting a simple cold. They have the potential to make me extremely ill and very likely threaten my life. As a consequence every year I'm given the seasonal influenza vaccination and I had a pneumonia vaccine back in 2001 that lasts ten years. Sadly there is no cure for the common cold so I'm always susceptible to catching it. This in turn makes me feel ultra concerned about hygiene. I was often making sure people washed their hands and covered their mouths and noses if they happen to cough or sneeze. Also I try and limit contact with outside carers and visitors who have colds and other illnesses; it's easier for them to stay away.

Gradually as the weeks passed my symptoms eased and I did indeed feel much better. My secretions had returned to their usual white colour as opposed to the horrid shade of yellow clogging up my chest. I was still having suction approximately two or three times a day but this was a vast improvement to the twenty or more times I was having it. My breathing had improved too and I was not struggling so much with it, requiring the ventilator only at night as per normal. My lungs didn't feel as they were in a metal jacket any longer but I always do dread the change of the seasons from winter to spring and from summer to autumn.

However all my worries about catching seasonal illnesses would make me feel like staying at home. This in turn meant I didn't want to socialise for fear of getting ill. Going out involved a military operation of arranging the suction machine, making sure the van was available, getting dressed, making sure I had a supply of catheters and gloves and taking my urine bottle. Also my parents would have to come with me to the venue incase I needed suction. There was also the fact that I needed to get back to go on my ventilator incase my lungs got overly tired.

By the time all of this was completed it would be hardly worth going out which meant I just didn't feel like it and would not bother. I didn't want to go out at all costs; I was and still am quite happy to stay at home.

An extra note on dressing, for you it might just consist of pulling your trousers up and buttoning a shirt but for me it's a bit more complicated. Firstly I'm hoisted on to my bed and I'm put in a near horizontal position (I can't lay flat due to my bad scoliosis) then my mother needs to move my legs into each trouser leg. This however tends to hurt my knees, hips and sometimes my spine with sharp stabbing pains that cannot be prevented. Next my mother pulls my trousers up toward my rear end as far as she can. Unfortunately I cannot roll on to my side anymore as the mini tracheotomy hurts my throat and sets me off coughing if I do. In order to pull my trousers up my mother raises the hoist above the bed (with me in it) and in a precarious sometimes worrying manoeuvre pulls my trousers up. Then it's over to the wheelchair to get comfortably seated.

This complex method of dressing really puts me off going out; I just don't want to be in pain every time I want to go somewhere. In general I avoid trousers and underwear but that doesn't mean I don't care about my modesty or decency. I usually sit on large *Tena* pads folded in half ever since I was put on diet pills, which sometimes acted like laxatives so often I couldn't make it in time. After I stopped taking them I still needed the pads due to how long it takes to get on to the toilet anyway. Next my legs are covered by two warm black fleece blankets that Sian made me, this keeps my dignity intact. I am extremely comfortable when I'm 'dressed' in this manner. Putting on tee shirts is a lot easier with a minimum amount of discomfort and I have loads of them in various colours and patterns. I have great difficulty getting into shirts, jumpers and waistcoats due to my arms hurting in any positions above my head, out to the side or behind my back so I tend to avoid them altogether.

# Age Nineteen

My nineteenth birthday was a fun fuelled day of games and the now traditional barbeque celebration. I seemed to be blessed with the weather most birthdays; it was another furnace of a day as pleasing warm sunshine draped over me. In the early afternoon we were all sitting outside sunbathing, Emma lying on a chairs' cushion reading one of her many favourite books, Sian listening to music all the while playing with her blonde hair, my father and I messing around with a cricket ball and my mother resting under a parasol. I was holding a small piece of wood which was light and straight, whilst my arm rested three inches in the air on a soft foam pad that Sian had made. I was trying to hit a red cricket ball that my father was gently throwing towards me.

With a swift action I just about managed to take a small swing at the ball; I could only move my hand an inch or two. The ball would just hit the wooden stick and drop like a stone onto my clear plastic wheelchair table; "Oooh nearly got it" I would say, frustrated. When I did manage a fractionally harder swing (which would make my whole body ache) I'd knock the ball, which bounced off my table and onto the scorched grass below. I would smile broadly when I finally made a proper connection; "Yes, get in there!" I would shout out happily. My father and I played our small makeshift game of cricket for a further hour until we were both well and truly tired as the hot sun poured down on us. Later I drove my wheelchair into the house craving an ice cold drink and some shade, waiting until that years' barbeque started.

My parents were in a frenzy getting food and makeshift seats ready for the evenings' festivities. I played with my presents and listened to some music on the family PC in my blue walled room. Guests started arriving soon after at around six o'clock in the evening. It was mostly family and family friends who attended including my uncle Alan a tall, dark haired crazy man who lights up any occasion and my aunty Deb a medium built blonde haired woman surrounded by many necklaces. My cousins Sarah a medium built light haired girl with a very interesting turn of phrase (due to her health issues) and Sean a tall blonde boy into all the latest fashions and gadgets. My aunties sister Jan, a very kind tall blonde lady who works in a hospital and her husband Rob a tall slightly balding dark haired man who always tells a few jokes. Also their son Matt a tall well built man who used to help me swim. Various other family members dropped by including my frail grandparents who had many interesting stories to tell.

I sat by a family friend liked by all called Emma who is a tallish black haired lady from a nearby town. She's so kind and pleasant towards me always greeting me with a friendly hug and wide smile. She gave me many cool presents over the years and I'm very grateful for them. She used to be a volunteer in my father's swimming club and often helped me during her time there. One memorable occasion at a previous barbeque, she was pouring my drinks for the evening topping up my *Vodka* and *Cola* and making me laugh. All this of course made me talk more and more into the fading evening. The next day I didn't remember too much but my jaw sure ached from my incessant yammering; I hope I'd made sense at the time!

The fun progressed for a few more hours as the pleasant summer smell of barbequed meat hung in the air. We played a quiz near the end of the night with my father acting as compare, drawing out any prizes from a mystery box whilst we laughed at our unusual answers. After the barbeque and whilst the guests were leaving, my parents and I talked over the evenings events reminiscing about all the funny moments we witnessed. I always enjoyed my barbeque birthdays up until it became impractical, as I find it impossible now to eat barbequed meat or any 'whole' food due to dysphagia (swallowing issues) caused by Duchenne's. Also the recent bad summers didn't help when planning an outdoor event, but then again there is always next year!

The big news story from around that time was the worrying S.A.R.S epidemic terrorizing Asia. It stood for Severe Acute Respiratory Syndrome which caused intense respiratory illness and was fatal in many cases. I was extremely frightened as it seemed inevitable (at the time) that a global pandemic would ensue. I was concerned as my immune system is extremely impaired and I had nearly died of respiratory problems back in 2001. I was willing it so hard not to come to Wales. Everyday the news got worse and worse with more cases developing and the growing spread of the virus reported ad infinitum in the media.

I know in reality there's nothing I can do to stop the spread of viruses like the current flu pandemic and back then S.A.R.S, but it didn't stop me worrying. Only the slightest of colds has the potential to seriously harm me so my fears were magnified a thousand times. In any case I would have to go to the hospital hoping that my respiratory consultant and respiratory team gave me the appropriate treatment early enough. Recently I have been given a preventative dose of antibiotics to use just incase I develop symptoms of an illness. One wrong move in regards to common illnesses and my health will suffer unnecessarily as I enter the so called terminal stages of Duchenne's.

Thankfully the WHO (World Health Organisation) and the affected countries managed to contain the outbreak around about the time of my birthday. My panic levels dropped significantly; watching twenty four hour news really didn't help with my previous anxiety. Bottling up fears and worries could make me feel run down, which in a cruel irony could lead to me developing an illness. It was this very cycle that partially led to me getting extremely ill in 2001 (the stress of exams and unmonitored respiratory function etc), so naturally I tried avoiding any sort of worry. Unfortunately that's an incredibly difficult and arduous task to undertake. Interestingly family life has a curious way of taking you're mind off things.

My eldest sister had some really important and wonderful news. After a romantic weekend away in Paris her long time boyfriend Ceri (a tall, quiet and slender man, liked by all of us, who often sported a trendy tee shirt) proposed on the top of the Eiffel tower. I was sitting in the lounge with my parents and Sian when the news broke; Emma stood there next to Ceri, with a huge smile on her face and a glorious little ring carefully perched upon her finger. My father quickly got a bottle of champagne from a nearby shop and we all toasted the splendid news well into the afternoon. My mother was smiling as she gave Emma a huge hug as well as offering sincere congratulations to Ceri. Sian and I were asking Ceri how he had proposed to Emma, "Did you go one knee Ceri?" we asked while laughing pleasantly.

Ceri told us the story about the events atop the Eiffel tower. He tried desperately to keep Emma in one place while he attempted to go on bended knee. Unfortunately my sister kept thinking he had lost something so she decided to move out of the way and try to help him find it! By now we were all laughing rapturously at this. Ceri continued with the story, he eventually managed to ask Emma for her hand by showing her the bright and sparkly engagement ring he had bought. Emma said "Yes" to that wonderful question as they stood in the cool Parisian air overlooking the tiny people scurrying about below. It must have looked like something out of all those romantic films you hear about, with the sun dipping below the horizon upon silhouetted lovers.

I was extremely happy that my sister was going to get married. I have always liked Ceri, we get on really well and he's a great guy; perfect for my eldest sister. It was now time for Emma, Ceri and our two families to prepare things for the wedding which was only twelve short months away. One of the many things that had to be prepared for was the issue of access so I could attend this most wonderful of occasions. Luckily the church Emma wanted to get married in was very accessible (I had been there many times). However finding an accessible venue for the wedding breakfast was an entirely different and somewhat daunting prospect.

Emma and my mother trawled many venues ranging from golf clubs to local hotels; a disused coal mine (which had function rooms in its visitor centre) and a beautiful manor house were also inspected. Every venue had to meet a certain number of requirements, including wide enough doorways and entrances, adequate disabled toilet facilities and enough parking room for my white *VW* van; obviously Emma had her own bridal requirements but I wasn't told about those. Whenever my mother and sister went to check out each of the venues they would take a tape measure and my wheelchair dimensions to size up the locations. I would hear stories of managers being grilled about access issues, I'm sure they weren't expecting all those questions!

Eventually and after much consideration and deliberation Emma chose Mais Manor as her venue for the wedding breakfast. To celebrate this fact we all had a meal in the Manor a few days later. We arrived at Mais Manor near the town of Blackwood on a beautiful afternoon just as the sun was beginning to drop. We entered through two ivy covered stone pillars into the pleasant lush grounds surrounded by many trees. The parking area was ideally sized for my van and the coaches that often frequented the Manor. The building itself looked to be Tudor styled with ornate grey stonework and large dark brown wooden windows; it overlooked a large grassy area with a gentle slope leading to some distant trees.

Once I was unloaded from the van I pressed a button to move my wheelchair forward using a modified *Playstation* control pad. It was made for me the previous year by ALAC (artificial limb and appliance centre), the inner workings were removed and new switches installed. I cannot use the usual wheelchair controls because my shoulder would slightly dislocate when trying to drive and my hands were getting too weak. To drive forward and backwards the 'X' and 'Square' buttons were used respectively. To steer I used the 'left' and 'right' buttons located on the *D-pad* (direction pad). I found it so easy to drive as I was using the same buttons whilst gaming all day on my *Playstation 2*. (Unfortunately I could only use this controller for a further two or so years until my hands became too deformed and further weakened, but for the time being it was an ingenious solution).

Inside Mais Manor we were greeted by an extremely helpful *Maitre de* who knew my mother and sister from their previous visits. We were shown into a lounge area with large plush leather armchairs pointed in the general direction of an extremely wide television. *Lancashire Lightning* was on that evening batting in a one day cricket match. We all enjoyed drinks while our table was being prepared, Sian and I had ice cold *Cola* in tall glasses with straws, Emma and Ceri had sparkling white wine along with my parents. The conversation centred on what I'd thought of the venue and later drifted on to the wedding plans. Eventually we were called in for our meal, we enjoyed the succulent beef that would be offered at the wedding breakfast (it's amusing how the meal after the wedding ceremony is called the *breakfast*).

After our wonderful tour of Mais Manor I was really pleased with the access and the disabled facilities were ideal. Over the next few weeks I still had to purchase a few items to make sure I was ready for the wedding. My main concern was finding a suitable shirt to wear, on the face of things this would seem like an extremely minor affair. In my case however sitting in a wheelchair all day as well as having scoliosis (a curved spine) meant I am an odd shape for clothing; I need a relatively small necked collar but a large amount of material for the bottom half around my waist. My parents tried everywhere to find a suitable shirt, they tried local stores, national chain stores and of course the ubiquitous internet stores.

In the end we found a store willing to make the necessary adjustments and within no time at all a crisp, smart white shirt arrived. After the usual tug of war match otherwise known as getting dressed, the shirt fitted quite well and to complete the look a purple cravat was added in line with the brides' wishes. I was happy that I would fit in with the rest of the men in my immediate family. Having to wear different clothes based on what my body allowed often made me feel a little left out. Back in school for instance I couldn't wear the smart shoes or even trainers that my peers were bragging about, this made conversation topics rather thin on the ground. The only clothes I can comfortably wear are tee shirts and the occasional polo shirt. Luckily the wedding day shirt fitted perfectly and more importantly I looked the part.

My final memories of the preparations were of endless hours enduring wedding programmes on the television. Whenever Emma wanted to know something relevant she would put the *Sky TV* on to watch such wonderful programmes as *Bridezilla*! I remember fondly arguing about this with Emma "Oh c'mon there MUST be something else on, Em!!" I would plead. We'd both laugh as I turned the television over with my environmental control, only for Emma to use the conventional remote to return to the wedding programming. In the end I always relented as the programmes generally lasted, at the most, an hour. I'm sure that after a few weeks of that I could name all the different types of dress and what would be an ideally suited cake for an Italian wedding! Luckily I'm an extremely patient and laid back guy, so I wasn't too bothered in the end.

August came around very quickly and I'm pretty sure everyone can remember the unbearable heat we had in 2003. To me it felt like the first steps of hell, breathing out hot air really wore me out. There was no escape from the oppression as temperatures often soared into the high twenties or thirties. I cannot move so this meant I rarely sweat but it was hot enough for even me to perspire. We bought two fans to try and cool ourselves (air conditioning isn't common in the UK); they worked to some extent but the heat still clawed at the back of my head. My bedroom was almost unbearable at night, it's usually warm (I have the heating on most of the time) but this was something entirely different.

I couldn't get over the extreme lethargy I felt after a whole day baking and sweating. I was looking forward to using my ventilator at night because I could get some much required rest. It had another benefit too, if whilst on the ventilator I moved my chin a few millimetres a cool blast of air would hit my clammy body and provide some instant cooling relief. I couldn't do this for too long as my lungs would be missing out on their rest. Another reason why venting air in this way isn't a great idea is because an alarm will sound indicating a loss of pressure. Not just any old alarm but a really loud high pitched whine that can really startle you (it has often woken the whole house!).

Thankfully relief came as the usual autumnal low pressure weather systems arrived; not a moment too soon in my opinion. The fans were quickly packed away and ironically my heating turned back on. I missed the sunshine (but not the extreme heat) as dark dreary rain filled afternoons quickly set in. Autumn and even winter days for me had become the same as any other. Since leaving school I was just stuck in the same routine always thinking there must be more than just *Playstation 2* games (even though I loved them) and the odd soiree into *Yahoo* games. The only thing that did change depressingly was the monster called Duchenne's which invades every fibre of my being. Most of the time I just tried to force the whole illness and its effects to the back of my mind; computer games obviously helped that. Also like I've said before my family always find a way of taking my mind off DMD and being an optimist can get you though the tough times.

Christmas time was the usual affair of excited build up and visits from the family. As usual my great aunty Rose, (a very prim and proper lady who has immaculate hair) and my great uncle Don, (a tall slender man who wears thick glasses) came over bearing gifts on Christmas Eve. It is one of the highlights of the year for us; the day always has a very familiar pattern. My great aunt and uncle usually arrive at about nine thirty in the evening carrying bright shiny bags full of presents for the whole family. My father would pour drinks, usually a spirit for my aunty and some non alcoholic *Elderflower* wine for my uncle. After the usual pleasantries we would all settle down in the lounge chairs to talk over the years events. I always occupy the same spot next to the armchair facing the television.

The ladies of the house will usually talk to Rose who would regale us with stories of dinner parties, news and her time working in a local factory. I loved the way she described the colourful stories which were full of intriguing and often extremely funny moments. The way Rose speaks reminds me of Margot from the 1970's series *The Good Life*, I'm certainly not the only one to say this she would often tell me. This always makes my parents and I smile. Although she's far more down to Earth than the very eccentric and snobbish Margot ever was.

Meanwhile the men of the house would listen to Don's stories of his time in the *Freemason's*, his stories of my parents wedding day and my favourite subject, his ability to make old style television and radio sets. It really fascinated me as my interest in science never swayed even though I failed that exam years ago. Talk of valves, transistors and crystal sets filled the air well into the evening. The rich noise of jovial conversation gently buzzed in the background; occasionally my father would laugh loudly at something Don would say. All the while I would focus in to different conversations briefly forgetting all about Duchenne's for one blissful night.

At about half past one in the morning we had exhausted all our conversational topics and would give our gifts to Rose and Don just before they left. They live on the other side of the village way up high on the mountain overlooking the pleasant greenness synonymous to the Welsh valleys. Once my great aunty and uncle left for home my mother and sisters would carefully place the presents under the multi-coloured Christmas tree. Next we would all wind our way up to bed; my mother stopping off in my room to put me into bed; once again using my ceiling hoist. With Christmas morning only a few hours away it was nearly impossible to sleep; even at age nineteen I was still excited about opening presents and seeing my family around the table.

When 2004 did eventually arrive it was back to my usual daily routine of computer games and the now weekly suctioning of my chest (I had gradually increased use because of the diseases progressive nature). Winters are always worse for my chest; almost yearly I would get seasonal illnesses (these have blighted my life ever since I was sixteen).

I would now like to go into the difficulties and challenges surrounding my type of paralysis. First of all my type of paralysis doesn't affect my sense of feeling as my spinal cord isn't damaged. Duchenne's induced paralysis is due to a total loss of muscle (as the muscle fibres die off and turn into connective tissue); which means I don't have the strength to move. Certain areas of my body still move but only to an extremely limited degree. For instance with two hands placed on my small computer mouse (my parents put my hands in the correct location) I have enough movement to move it a centimetre or two. However my fingers do not move much at all, only one thumb has enough strength to push the light mouse buttons. With the pointer speed set to maximum I can just about manage to operate a computer. Also I can barely move my feet, I can raise my heel up in the air by a half centimetre but not forward, backward or from side to side. Every other part of my body cannot move so I describe myself as ninety nine percent paralysed or very much like a quadriplegic (in 2004 I could move my hands and fingers slightly more but DMD always gets progressively worse).

Incase you're having difficulty imagining this state of affairs try to think of it like this. Imagine you're sitting on a chair, and then imagine your legs and arms are chained tightly into place. Next your hands are taped into fist shapes leaving a thumb free on your right hand to click (your thumb cannot be fully straitened either). Your spine is pushed forward and to the side at the same time and a huge concrete weight is balanced on your head. Your head is resting on a headrest due to the aforementioned concrete weight and there's an iron weight surrounding your chest making breathing hard. Lastly (in my case) there's a small hole in your throat with a plastic tube fitted in there. I know it sounds harsh but hopefully this gives you a brief insight into my type of paralysis and condition.

Certainly the most infuriating part of being paralysed and being able to feel is when something irritates my skin. For instance when I get an itch on my leg, it's so irritating it almost feels like a stinging pain. Chinese water torture has got nothing on an itch you cannot scratch. The only way I avoid going crazy is to think of another part of my foot or leg that isn't itching and concentrate on that. In time and with much effort the itch seems to disappear; if it's too unbearable I'll ask my mother to scratch my leg. It's extremely difficult however to direct my mother to the exact spot; I just say "Up a bit" or "Down a bit". The relief once the spot has been located is overwhelming that is, until the next irritant comes along.

Another personally annoying part of paralysis is not being able to help out around the house. For instance I'd love to make my parents a cup of tea but boiling a kettle and pouring the liquid out is an impossible dream at the moment. Washing and dressing my self would be an amazing independence boost too but I have had become used to being dressed by others. I grew up with my condition always getting worse so things like being dressed never really bothered me. Although it is hard you do get used to it in the end; I'm constantly redefining my image of "normal". Helping out with chores is also difficult, I'd love to be able to wash the car and tidy my room (I'm assuming most people would run away screaming from that). To keep my sanity intact however I just concentrate on what I can do; internet browsing and shopping for my parents is one of the tasks I can perform.

It was around this time that I started becoming increasingly isolated in my bedroom. I was basically living in there. I suppose what drove me upstairs was a mixture of fear about illnesses and not having much to do downstairs. I had no friends to speak of so I didn't even have anyone to ring and chat with. I would play the *Playstation 2* for hours up until five in the afternoon and then I'd move on to the family PC after my evening meal. Often I'd end up sitting in the dark staring at a bright computer screen whilst playing *Yahoo* Pool. I'd notice the clock tick over to eleven and finally decide to make an appearance downstairs. I wasn't particularly depressed or upset at the time I was just trying to avoid boredom and keep my brain occupied through the lonely days. It's great talking to my mother and thankfully we get on very well, but I felt lonely even though I was surrounded by my family and the occasional doctor or nurse.

I'd like to explain what my blue walled bedroom actually looks like (as I have mentioned it fairly often). As I've mentioned before the extension at the back of my house contains my through-floor lift. After the brief journey between floors I enter and am immediately confronted by the 'back' room of my bedroom. The extension created this space meaning my room is essentially two different areas merged together. There is quite a lot of space but it quickly gets filled. As I was saying the back is where I exit my lift, on the wall that used to be the exterior of the house there are three long shelves. The top shelf holds some small travelling cases and my father's woodworking router. The second shelf holds some CD's and office supplies such as printer paper and ink cartridges. The third and final shelf houses some of my medical supplies namely my suction gloves.

On my left is the rear bedroom window which overlooks our small garden. There's plenty of room for my wheelchair to turn; this really makes things a whole lot easier. Under the third shelf lie the rest of my large medical supplies such as boxes of suction catheters and a box of *Tena* pads used to cover my bed and wheelchair. Only recently do I store my mobile hoist by the window, it creates a better space in our living room (where it used to reside). On the right are pictures of my day with former Prime Minister Sir John Major with our grinning faces beaming down from the wall. Next I pass through the old exterior wall into the 'front' room; you can see how big the original walls are as there's a good two foot thickness visible.

In the 'front' room there's a radiator on the right coloured in the deep blue paint I've had in my room for many years. On the left is my single occupancy hospital bed that is adjustable (the feet and head parts move). Sadly there isn't a king size version, if I had a girlfriend we'd literally have to be 'intimate' just to get in! Back on the right there's a moveable desk which used to house my *Playstation 2* until heartbreakingly I had to sell it in 2005. By the door I have a wall mounted cabinet full of ventilator supplies and some shelves housing my collection of antique pocket watches. Lastly hanging over the foot of my bed is a small LCD screen which I sometimes use for watching television. It's a good sized double room that really suits my needs, although sometimes it feels like an extension to a hospital ward given all the supplies I have!

The final thing I remember about being nineteen was a quite alarming deterioration in my chewing and swallowing. One sunny morning I tried eating some fruit whilst my father fed me, I began chewing but as soon as the small food bits where ready to be swallowed, I just couldn't activate my swallowing mechanism. I tried everything, smaller chunks of fruit, chewing harder and even psyching myself up. However nothing worked and I became increasingly distressed. I even had to spit the bits out that I couldn't swallow, this was extremely scary and I felt very embarrassed. If I was careful there were certain foods I could eat but even then I still had to spit the odd hard particle out. As you can imagine this restricted my diet immensely and unbeknownst to me I slowly began to lose weight.

Not that any of this was monitored by a neuromuscular consultant. I hadn't then been to a specialist for approximately ten years (I still haven't seen one). Since professor Sibert retired from his muscle clinic in the mid nineties, the NHS didn't appoint a replacement and shamefully as a result services have steadily declined into nothing. For instance there was no guidance from a specialist when my scoliosis was left uncorrected. This meant my spine has further curved quite severely and that in turn is affecting my breathing. This leads me on to the lack of respiratory monitoring I received between the ages of ten and sixteen. As you've previously read I developed pneumonia and required three stays in intensive care during 2001 because of this lack of monitoring.

Physiotherapy stopped at age sixteen after leaving school and this has meant my contractures have got a lot worse. It's impossible to straighten my fingers, trying to do so will cause me a lot of pain and could break a bone. Interestingly because I received so few care packages from the social services my social worker 'closed' the case on me. I'd be happy with that if only my disease had miraculously disappeared overnight! This lack of care really makes me feel forgotten about. Why is this happening to me? Why isn't my deadly disease taken seriously? These two questions often come to mind and I have no obvious answers to give.

The only consultant I was visiting (on a six monthly basis) was my respiratory specialist. They have no specific DMD credentials just a special interest in the condition. I now have my breathing monitored by a very competent team and I'm extremely grateful of the emergency care they gave me in 2001. Although their grasp on my other medical conditions is limited; as naturally they only concentrate on one part of my body. I do wish however that a muscle specialist would guide me and the team into further possible preventative solutions, and not the 'reactionary' medicine I always seem to get.

I now know that I should be getting a multi-disciplined care approach (with eight or so neuromuscular specialist doctors and nurses), which has proven very successful in Newcastle and London in improving life expectancy into the thirties. Where as at the moment in Wales the average life expectancy is an alarming nineteen, somehow I have made it past that despite the non existent care I am currently enduring. Recently I've been campaigning to change this shocking and unfair treatment existent in Wales (much more on this in subsequent chapters).

# *Age Twenty*

For the first time I can remember it rained on my birthday. Our usual barbeque only had a few guests' mainly immediate family. There was Uncle Alan, Aunty Deb and my cousins along with Sian, Emma, Ceri and my parents. The rain was coming down quite heavily. The day before Alan and my father had put up a blue tarpaulin in the Garden. I drove my wheelchair roughly over the back door threshold and rode under the tarp listening to the drops patter playfully on the plastic. It was strange sitting under the plastic as everything took on a blue hue, our voices were echoing around the small covered area. Ceri was attending to the barbeque with his friend Phil, an average height man with a heart of gold. The smells of the barbeque quickly filled the area; they managed to light it despite the rain. It was particularly hard taking in the smells of the delicious meat all the while knowing I couldn't eat any of it. However I never let it bother me and was busily joking with Alan by the time everything was cooked.

I had to have my dinner before the event; I struggled to swallow the soft potato fritters I usually ate. At least the tomato ketchup tasted superb you can't beat *Heinz* in my opinion. The conversation stayed firmly on Emma's wedding by now only a mere month away. I didn't feel like my birthday on that wet dreary day. I suppose the magic just disappears when you never know what you want to get. Computer games were getting harder to play so my gift choices dwindled, it was around this time I developed my passion for all things collectable including watches. At least with watches all you need to do is look at them and not handle them. I love the perfection and simplicity of time, watching the hands creep silently across the dial. I received a very simple gold pocket watch that birthday which still hangs happily in my room.

The special day quickly arrived. August the twentieth 2004 was the day my eldest sister Emma got married. Luckily the weather was dry but low grey clouds hugged the rooftops. Emma lived two doors away at the time. She got up early to get pampered by the hair dresser and to put on her wonderful dress. It was a long white figure hugging dress with pretty little flowers adorning the front. Sian and my mother also took turns getting preened by the hairdresser; although I'm told she was very slow! I was soundly asleep on my ventilator at the time waiting for my nine o'clock wake up call. I had many mixed dreams of what was about to happen that day. I was so excited and nervous for my sister and most importantly extremely happy for her.

Nine o'clock arrived soon enough and my mother burst into my room ready to help me go downstairs. My grey sling was connected to the overhead hoist and carefully I was manoeuvred above my wheelchair and gently lowered in. Next I quickly drove into my grey metal through-floor lift and one minute later I arrived on the ground floor. I drove past the bathroom and on into the kitchen where my father had breakfast waiting. I struggled to eat my spaghetti hoops but twenty minutes later I was finished and ready for a wash. I pressed the buttons on my modified *Playstation* control pad and quickly zoomed into the bathroom. My mother had a hot flannel waiting to wash my face with, which was flushed from a night on the ventilator. She had to carefully avoid rubbing the bridge of my nose because of the soreness.

Once my mother finished washing me, I had to go straight back upstairs into my room. Whilst there my mother once again hoisted me back into bed. I was laid on to my back and my sling was moved out the way. My mother skilfully placed each of my legs into my underwear and the black trousers I had to wear for the day. They were pulled up as far as they could be. Next the sling was moved back into place and attached to the hoist. I was hoisted up above the bed and my mother pulled my trousers and boxer shorts up as far as she could manage; all the while the hoist would swing.

After my dressing aerobatics it was back into my wheelchair where my crisp white shirt was put on. I was then escorted to the lift and again one minute later arrived at the ground floor. I drove into the lounge and parked in my usual spot facing the television. I started talking to a family relative called Lloyd who was staying with us for the wedding. He is a tall man with stylish hair and always approachable. We talked about the upcoming wedding ceremony and his special interest in photography. Every now and then his brown haired girlfriend Ellie would walk past either doing her hair or adjusting her outfit. We were all waiting for a lift to the church which was being provided by my Aunties brother in law Robert. The well built slightly balding man who attended a few of my birthday barbeques.

Robert arrived at around eleven thirty with his wife Jan in tow. I drove my wheelchair around the back of the house and out to the front. Once out the front I waited for my white *VW* van to be opened and its side mounted lift made ready for me. I edged back onto the lift and was raised up level with the vans' floor. I backed into my spot and the wheelchair was clamped in and the red safety seatbelt placed around my waist. Next Lloyd, Ellie and my mother got in and took their seats. Finally Rob put the lift into its travelling position and then started the vans throaty engine. The journey was very short as we passed over the bridge to the 'other' side of the village and up a few steep hills towards the church.

We arrived outside the large church and we were all unloaded onto a very bumpy pavement. I trundled and bounced my way towards the iron gates all the while trying to avoid the wedding video cameraman. I'm very shy about appearing in videos and I've only recently tried to overcome this. I quickly drove into the church itself and talked to some very familiar people, including my uncle Alan and a few distant relatives. I was parked in a space next to my mother up front near the altar. Soon enough the beautiful wedding car arrived and Emma got out with her train flowing majestically behind. Sian and Bethan (Emma's best friend), a lovely tall blonde lady, were bridesmaids for the day wearing attractive lilac dresses. Bethan's first daughter Ffion was the flower girl wearing a similarly coloured dress to her mother.

The wedding march started up on the church organ and in walked Emma smiling broadly whilst Sian and Bethan escorted her up the aisle. Ffion skipped merrily behind them with a pleasant smile on her bright little face. Ceri was standing up front not far from me in his fine wedding suit, waiting for his perfect bride to arrive at his arm. My father met Emma halfway up the aisle so he could give her away as is wedding tradition. A few minutes later the church fell silent and the vicar began the service. The vows were read out and recited nervously by the happy couple. I felt so happy for my eldest sister on her special day. Finally Ceri was allowed to kiss the bride, to which everyone clapped and gasped in pleasure. Shortly after Emma and Ceri disappeared into a side room where they signed all the necessary paperwork; the guests and I waited in our seats talking.

After what seemed like twenty minutes the newlyweds came back out of the side room looking very pleased. They quickly walked down the aisle towards the exit at the rear of the church as beautiful organ music played. Shortly after they disappeared into their chauffer driven car and headed to Mais Manor. Next all the assembled guests headed toward their coach which was waiting noisily in the street. My mother, Lloyd and Ellie accompanied me once again to the van where Robert and his wife Jan were waiting. I backed onto the lift and was raised into the van where my chair was reclamped and the red belt reattached. We then slowly proceeded toward the manor situated near the town of Blackwood. The journey passed really quickly as we talked over the wedding ceremony with Robert and Jan.

It wasn't long before we were passing through the same ivy covered gates we had seen the year before. We actually arrived before the coach even though we set off later. Apparently there was uproar on the coach after it got delayed going the long way round; my Uncle didn't want to miss the free bar! My family and I still laugh about that every year. My uncle persuaded my father to extend the free bar and things settled down fairly quickly. A few minutes later everyone arrived and poured out of the coach. I drove over to meet my cousin and Sian, we were all handed a buck's fizz (Orange juice and Champagne) or Champagne depending on our preferences. My mother held a cold tasty buck's fizz up to my lips and I gratefully knocked it back.

While the bride and groom were outside having their professional photos taken we all proceeded to the lounge inside the manor. I've never seen so many drinks bought in such a short time; everyone was certainly making the most of the free bar! I was sat by a few of my aunties who were busily chain smoking; it wasn't long until I moved as the smoke started to choke me. After about twenty minutes we were all called back outside for photographs; we were led out into an unseasonably chilly August afternoon. It was quite hazy by now as the dark clouds lifted and broke up a little above us. My jaw started aching after all my talking and the constant smiling everyone seems to do on a wedding day. We were grouped into all sorts of family ensembles with me being quite prominent in many of the photos. It was turning into a thoroughly enjoyable afternoon.

The evening quickly set upon us and we all retreated into the manor houses' function room. We all settled down at our designated tables. I was heaved and pushed up a very steep ramp so I could join the top table near Emma and our family. In no time at all the meals were brought out, beef or fish on the menu. I didn't have any meat as I could only just about manage the soft vegetables. It was delicious and quieted our rumbling stomachs; ice cold *Cola* and Wine were a great addition to the fare. An hour later after all the plates were cleared away, the tall *maitre de* approached the table nearest me and began tapping loudly with an auctioneer's gavel. He announced the start of the wedding speeches.

The most captivating speech came from the best man who made everyone rock with laughter that evening. His name was Hywel, a short spiky haired man who looked very nervous while delivering his monologue. He came out with all sorts of comments, some funny and some serious but a lot were very touching. By the end we were all laughed out and give him a huge round of applause as he filed back to his seat. My father's speech was very interesting, with the odd funny cherished moment thrown in too. Often this would make Ceri and Emma blush but it was all done in good humour. I could tell by the way he was talking how proud of Emma he was. It was great to listen too. As a final surprise he read out a poem written by Bethan; Emma's best friend.

The funniest speech was from Uncle Alan, who by now was very merry after the exploits of the free bar. His speech was full of humour and jest but underneath all that was a touching sincerity. In one funny moment he said "...I've been planning Emma's life ever since she met Ceri..." we all laughed at that. He continued "...I'm sure it won't be long until she has the first of many kids!" To which Emma started to shake her head in a sort "as if" gesture. His final act was to give out a special joke gift to Ceri (Alan's tradition for family weddings). He gave him a blow up hammer and a bob the builder helmet because of the building mishaps Ceri had whilst doing up his first house.

The evening for me quickly came to end at around seven when I was driven home by Robert. I was getting tired by then so we had the rest bite carers coming in so my mother could attend the rest of the wedding night. I thoroughly enjoyed the day and have taken away fantastic memories that are always a comfort to me on particularly hard days, which often accompany Duchenne's. I told the carers all about the fantastic day I had but the rest of the night was a blur until my parents came home. It wasn't long until I was helped into bed by my mother all the while she regaled me with stories of the disco and conversations she had. The moment my head hit the pillow I fell into a deep sleep and dreamed about whether I'd have my own wedding some day.

Autumn soon arrived with its usual gales and stormy weather battering the country. It signalled a big change for me in terms of what I was able to do during the day. Increasingly I was finding it very difficult to play on my beloved *Playstation 2*. My hands could barely move, my fingers were very stiff and it would take me a long time just to press start. Pressing select was nigh on impossible and I was exhausted after a few hours gaming. In no time at all I couldn't use the games console whatsoever and it had to be sold. I was unashamedly heartbroken by this seemingly trivial event. I would never again be able to play football or drive a virtual supercar on my favourite driving game. The saying "As one door closes another opens" seemed very apt in what was to come.

What stopped me going insane with boredom was the switch to using our family desktop computer full time. In the beginning of my adventure into a new world of *Windows XP*, I just played solitaire and listened to my growing collection of music. I'm into trance, dance, some alternative genres and indie; my favourite indie rock band is the *Stereophonics*. Once solitaire began to lose its novelty factor I began exploring our recently installed broadband internet. I started off not knowing how the net worked but within no time at all I was totally up to speed. I visited loads of websites, discovering a multitude of information about my disease and playing the ever ubiquitous games. I naturally hovered around *Yahoo*'s main site because that was my default homepage. I enjoyed checking out the news and playing all sorts of card games. I also frequented *Amazon* looking for books and computer equipment.

I continued all this fun and entertainment well into the January of 2005. During that time I was getting quite bored sitting downstairs. I felt naked without the computer in he evening and television was getting all too tedious for me. I needed a solution quickly, save for bringing the desktop computer down with me, I was all out of ideas. By March however I found the answer to my problems and that was a top of the range laptop my father bought me via a charitable organisation. Originally my mother thought me having a laptop was an extravagant luxury but soon enough she realised how much I enjoyed using it. Everyday had a new familiar pattern to it, in the morning I'd use the family desktop until around five in the afternoon and then switch to my laptop downstairs until it was time to sleep.

Quickly enough I discovered *MSN* messenger sitting on the computers' desktop and I was intrigued by the idea of real time conversations over the internet. I opened the program and discovered that there was no one to talk too it seems you need friends first. I wracked my brain trying to locate someone to talk too. I solved that problem after listening to my sister Emma; remembering her saying something about chat rooms. Immediately I rushed over to a search engine and typed in 'chat rooms'. I found literally millions of hits and became totally confused as to which one to visit. I bit the bullet so to speak and choose a seemingly professional site. It warned the now usual warning about not putting up personal information or giving out credit card details. I was fine with all that and soon enough clicked the brightly coloured *ENTER* button.

It was daunting at first and often confusing to see my unique ID sprouted out as my name. Quickly it became second nature. I had loads of fun joining in crazy conversations about bar rooms and alien landings. You just never know what is coming next in a chat room and I just rolled with the flow. I didn't have to be disabled there as I could type anything my mind wanted. If I want to pretend I was an athlete, I could, or if I pretend to make the tea or pass someone a virtual beer I can do that too. It's a perfect escape from an often cruel world and equally cruel disease. Personally I didn't want to hide behind a false persona; soon enough my true self started to come through. Even though I was being myself I felt no-one judging me, perhaps they thought this was another persona.

In no time at all I became quite friendly with two or three of the regular chatters. We were talking on *MSN* messenger most nights and would often chat well into the small hours of the night. I carried on like this over the next couple of weeks. I thought I've got this chat room business down to a tee and began moving around to other chat rooms. It wasn't the same as the first time around but indeed I found talking to people really interesting. It is difficult to sift out the genuine people from the cruel and weird but I thought I was doing well so far. That's when things took an unfortunate turn for the worse. My problems all started in the very first chat room I'd found.

Apparently I made a chat room faux pas by asking another member if she had just received a phone call from one of my new friends; with whom I was chatting on *MSN* messenger. I was immediately bombarded by this other member who verbally (typed out of course) abused me. I said "I'm sorry! I hadn't realised what I'd said was so wrong and I'm relatively new to chat rooms". However she continued her tirade at me and I began to feel threatened. Inevitably I cracked under the pressure by issuing a minor swear word and telling her to shut up. Meanwhile I contacted the friend on *MSN* messenger to tell him what was being said, but he basically backed the other persons view. It transpired that they were talking about me behind my back and I felt like a complete fool having to fight back red hot tears.

After I told this person to "shut up" she immediately kicked me out of the room and banned me for twenty four hours. It turned out this person was an administrator too. My so called *MSN* messenger friend told me "you shouldn't have said [expletive] to an admin". I'd never got in any sort of trouble before so I became worried and began to feel sick. I apologized profusely to the only other admin I could find at the time who was in the chat rooms sister site. She seemed unconcerned and reassured me that it wasn't a major thing I had done. That put my mind at ease and I felt a lot calmer. I made a decision that night to never return to that particular site ever again. It would make me feel awkward and fearful of other possible bans for things I didn't know I was doing. For the time being I left all things chat related behind until my confidence returned.

I knew one site that didn't make me feel uncomfortable or awkward and that was *Yahoo! Games*. I wanted to dedicate myself to one particular game instead of the usual trawling around I did on other games' websites. I remembered from a previous year my love of pool and snooker games and it wasn't long until I found a suitable 'room' to play in. A room is basically a central place which has up to two hundred and fifty tables and a small chat bar. My favourite pool game is American Eight ball and the room I first entered was named after a popular song sung by Queen. I saw the chat bar and decided not to talk to anyone as I was still weary of offending someone. Instead I'd quickly create a table and play all and sundry while keeping a watchful eye on the main chat bar. Perhaps I could learn the proper internet etiquette (or netiquette) from the regular pool goers I see in the room.

Every so often an advert would flash up in the chat bar promising fun times if you joined an online pool league. I was intrigued by this and decided to check out the leagues' website to see what all the commotion was about. I saw a list of rules aimed at keeping a friendly family atmosphere and found them most agreeable. Also I found a vast variety of different pool games we could play without leaving the room. Before committing myself to sign up I decided to talk (type) to the person who kept advertising this fun league. I'd seen this person chatting to others, talking with respect and always willing to help out the new guy or girl who had recently joined. For some reason I decided to put off joining for a few more days, as I suspect my anxiety about chat rooms was still lingering in the back of my mind.

Eventually I swallowed my fears and began typing out my hellos to everyone in the room. The person who had been advertising quickly greeted me and introduced herself as Demi. At first and to my great embarrassment I thought Demi was a guy! There were plenty of comical moments where our wires crossed but after seeing other members call her "hun" short for honey, finally the penny dropped. Rather sheepishly I began referring to Demi in the correct manner. As ever Demi handled it in her usual cooperative and unflustered way. After all the mix ups I finally got around to talking about the league. Demi cheerfully told me all the up sides and everyone else seemed so welcoming that I simply couldn't refuse.

I joined within an hour of Demi's cheerful and bright explanation of the league. The signup procedure baffled me but with a little help from the members and Demi I was in. How this particular league works was thus, you could play games with other members called 'leagues' abbreviated 'lgs'. You can win ranking points with every victory and lose points with every defeat. However most members preferred to play pool tournaments abbreviated 'trnys', which could earn you tokens. Theses tokens called bux are redeemable for prizes. Every tournament was hosted by a volunteer member who assumed the title of 'Tournament Director' or TD. Demi was an Admin in the league who ran tournaments, looked after matters of discipline and helped train new TDs.

Everyday I had something to get up for and put most Duchenne related problems to the back of my mind. There's a great camaraderie built up whilst being a league member so much so that all the regulars knew my name. Likewise I knew theirs too. The welcomes when I came in the room often took five minutes as everybody would join in. We would talk about our pool ratings, how our families were and when was the next tournament coming up. I would type for hours without thinking of the dull arm ache I always seemed to get. It was so uplifting talking to other people (for years I felt my isolation growing) now I felt part of something bigger. Demi was steadfastly there working all hours entertaining the masses with all the different games of pool.

I quickly became firm friends with Demi and we still are to this day. Everyone in the league used *Yahoo!* Messenger for private and fun conversations. Naturally at first I was a little wary of using the messenger after my tribulations with *MSN*, but as I considered these people proper friends (most still are) my hesitation didn't last long. Demi was one of the first I invited to become messenger friends and as she was British we already had something in common. More and more people invited me including Demi's partner who is a really good bloke from the United States. Demi and I confided in each other many things that never made the lobby (chat bar) as our trust grew. It's extremely difficult to gain some ones trust on the internet as you need to be ever vigilant, but I'd found a real friend in Demi.

As the hot sultry June days approached I was getting more and more curious about the role of Tournament Director. The TDs seemed to work together like a well oiled machine and were a closely nit team of staff. Demi would often say how easy it was to become a TD but warned that you needed the dedication to stick at it. I was always saying "Am I good enough to be a TD Demi?" to which she would answer "you're here everyday Ian and you know everyone so you seem well suited." That would set my mind racing with thoughts of whether I really was cut out to host tournaments. After all this would be my first ever 'job' albeit a voluntary unpaid position so I was nervous of clicking on that application form.

One warm night I decided I'd had enough of waiting and thinking about it. I filled out the brief form which asked when I was free. It so happened that most of my day was free; it was going to be so much fun being responsible for hosting tournaments in the league. Demi was the one who trained me in all my duties, including the running of tournaments and how to deal with any disputes that might erupt. In the event of rule breaking, TDs were expected to take screen shots of the offensive comments etc and report them back to the Admins. In no time at all I was well into my stride as one of the staff.

Most members liked me and I tried to be as approachable as I could. You'd get the jokers who would try it on but on the whole I managed quite well. Due to my strict rule following (I was aiming to keep a friendly inoffensive atmosphere), a few of the regulars nicknamed me Mr Censor! This made me smile but my approach certainly kept the arguing to a minimum. I started putting in long hours hosting many tournaments and getting new members to join up. It was amazing being able to do this despite having a disease that paralyses me.

# Age Twenty One

My twenty-first birthday was the last of our family barbeques; the planning involved and my continuing difficulty eating really started making things awkward. I was just happy to have quieter birthdays in, with the odd drink thrown in of course! Turning twenty one signalled a British tradition of receiving the "key to the door". Ironically and amusingly I've never been able to reach the front door let alone insert a key; it's the thought that counts. I remember receiving quite a few ceremonial keys on the morning of the fourteenth. My parents' key came with a pint glass so that made it even better. Shame I'm not a big drinker, I find the bitter after taste of alcohol hard to appreciate but I'm up for trying most things. The first beverage the glass held was my favourite soft drink *Pepsi Max*; I much prefer the pleasing ice cold caramel-like taste it delivers.

A golden sun heated the garden pleasantly while all the guests milled around grabbing toasted chicken wings and all manner of accompaniments. A gentle breeze caressed our green tablecloth and it would often flap up in the odd gust. I had my usual dinner of soft potato fritters and just managed to get some breaded fish down before the guests arrived. All accompanied with as you've probably guessed; some more *Pepsi Max*. It was a smaller family gathering, again, Uncle Alan, Aunty Deb and my cousins Sean and Sarah came over. Also Sian and her friends Reanna (a tall lady with dark hair and glasses) and Rebecca (a shorter dark haired lady who loves chicken) attended. Ceri and Emma came over from their house bearing salad and vegetarian alternatives because Emma had always been a vegetarian. A school video showing an abattoir had put her right off meat, which was highly understandable!

With a hat flopping over my eyes I sat covered in blankets gently slurping some Vodka and *Coke*. The night quickly started to draw in as my birthday always made me think of summer's end. I feel the cold terribly when sat outside (I'm sure I don't have any blood!) so I try to get my whole body covered. All you can see is my head floating above my black blankets. Again our family friend Emma popped in; her usual high spirits always make a party that extra bit fun. I was sitting next to her laughing and joking until my jaw started to ache; as usual the alcohol made me talk an excessive amount. I really felt it the day after but it's one of those things you get used to with muscle weakness.

We finished the evening watching midges cluster around a bright halogen lamp my dad hired for the day. My eyes felt really heavy by the time we got back inside the house. Still my family and I continued on talking and drinking soft drinks well past two in the morning. Only an hour or two earlier had the last guest filtered out of our garden to get some well earned rest. "It was a great barbeque ... this year Mam, it was great to see ... everyone" I slurred out in my usual Welsh accent. After finishing up the last dregs of my final *Pepsi Max*, I asked my mother to switch my chair on and in next to no time I was being hoisted into bed. It wasn't at all long until I drifted off to a largely dream free and fulfilled sleep.

As predicted by Uncle Alan, Emma was indeed pregnant less than a year after her wedding day. By August she was already three months pregnant and starting to show. For some reason I was very excited about this news, I always thought sisters getting pregnant was a thing for television films. I think babies are the coolest little bundles of cuteness you could ever wish for. Emma got me looking on the internet finding pregnancy tips and forcing me to endure endless visits to the *Mothercare* website. Goodness knows what she was putting Ceri through! My mother was busily knitting a neutrally coloured matinee coat as Emma didn't want to know the sex of her unborn child.

Every week Emma would ask me what she should be doing and how big the foetus was; this based on the web surfing I was doing for her. "Oooh I'd say Alfie is about the size of a grapefruit by now Em!" I would excitedly tell her. I don't know who was more excited, me, Emma, Ceri or my mother, it was definitely a close call there. We nicknamed the growing unborn baby Alfie and we would all ask how he/she was doing whenever Emma popped over to the house. I have no idea where we got the nickname from but it really seemed to fit. Maybe we got it from Michael Caine's character from the film of the same name but that's just a guess.

As October gently slid into November and the trees started to turn Emma was finding it more difficult to walk around; but she had that glow you often read about. Ceri was busily working for a small supermarket whilst also finishing up their house which was bijou to say the least. He was hoping Emma had a boy but he was so happy for her that obviously it wasn't an issue. He was brilliant with Emma all the way through her pregnancy and took good care of her. If Emma was feeling bored or wanted a cup of tea and a chat she'd only have to waddle past a few houses to see me and our mother. Sian was going back and for from various jobs trying to find a career that suited her. It's good having Sian around as we are of a similar age, so there's always plenty to talk about. We were both excited for Emma and would often talk about baby presents and how much we'd spoil the little one.

My father was so pleased to hear he was going to be a granddad that he couldn't wait to tell everyone at his office. He would often reminisce about taking me to *Toys R Us* when I was a young child; so I could tell he was excited. It had been quite awhile since any children had graced our house and this was definitely going to change things! My mother was busily trying to make sure Emma had all the things she needed, including a buggy, car seat, Moses basket and many more items that a baby could possibly need! At first my mother kept saying "Ah I'm too young to be a granny" so she decided that the future child should call her Nana. Emma's mother in law decided that she would like to be called gran, so that made things a lot easier and hopefully less confusing for the future little one.

As I've said before I was very pleased for Emma and couldn't wait till my niece or nephew was born. Also at the back of my mind were thoughts about my own parental desires to have children. I want one day to become a father and to be called dad myself. There are lots of barriers associated with relationships anyway so the added difficultly of DMD doesn't make things any easier. Finding girlfriends while stuck indoors is very difficult, my only hope being the internet; but you have got to be careful using that. Sex feels like a very distant dream for me but I still have these parenting desires floating in my head. This is probably an entirely normal human instinct; although it's very strange to be thinking of that whilst my sister was the one actually having a child.

As a distraction to keep my mind occupied I would spend the odd night surfing around *Amazon*. I'd search around the book section seeing if there was something that caught my imagination. I'm really into science fiction, crime fiction and the odd thriller. For a change though I decided to check out the computer software section. After clicking through about twelve pages of boring database software I came across a brightly coloured picture. The photograph showed a box with a multicoloured train drawn on it. It was in the style of a wooden toy, but you could definitely tell it was drawn. I glanced over to the description and saw the product was called *Corel Draw*. I was absolutely intrigued and kept getting drawn (no pun intended) back to the train and imagining myself designing it.

I felt something building inside me which I can only assume now was a remembrance of my previous school art exploits. I thought my drawing days were long over, but here in front of me on the screen was proof that I could now draw on the computer! I was so excited that I was busily telling my parents all evening about the program I'd found. My mother said "If you want it love just order it and give it a try" in her usual happy brogue. Whereas my father kept asking "What do you like about it and are you sure you can use your mouse with it?" I would answer those questions with "I love the fact that I can draw or paint and yes it only requires a mouse".

That satisfied my parents who said to order it when I was ready. However in a slight twist, whilst on the software pages I came across an even better art program. It was called *Corel Painter IX* and featured a very strange drawing of a hand with many fingers on the box. It was most definitely eye catching and I became even more excited than when I first found *Corel Draw*. As my father was sitting nearby I quickly showed him the new art creating software and we bought it there and then. It was quite pricey but my father helped me out with the cost and soon enough we had a confirmation email sitting in our inbox. It was a terribly long wait checking with my mother everyday to see if we had any large post!

After the longest three weeks I can remember it finally arrived on our doorstep. It was a typical miserable winter's day somewhat brightened by the arrival of a giant purple box. It had travelled from a far flung American state but looked no worse for wear. My mother carefully opened the folded box under my watchful eye and guidance. She unfurled the instructions and laid them out in front of me; this was impossible for me to do because of my severely weakened and deformed hands. I quickly established how easy it was to install and located the CD and registration details. In no time at all I had the installation screen flashing on my laptop; a bright green progress bar was slowly counting down in front of me.

Once it was loaded I opened the program and started to read the online instructions I was directed too. It all went way over my head and I couldn't tell a paintbrush from a colour palette. I decided to just jump in and click on every drop down menu box and like a typical male I ignored the instructions. After a day or two I'd managed to open a new painter document and found a basic digital oil-paint brush to use. My early scribbles and sploshes were just aimed at getting a feel for paintbrush speeds and sizes. I don't recall what my very first painting looked like but I did show it to my father one dark winters evening. However I do remember the first painting I did for a friend (crudely drawn by my current standards) which featured a mysterious woman walking down a desert road.

Finding inspiration to come up with a new painting was very difficult at first. As my skills were new and fresh I would often get frustrated if my attempts wouldn't match my visions. I also had great trouble concentrating on my artwork as other things kept getting in the way; such as checking emails, doing some shopping and my addiction to online pool! Like a child who gets bored I decided to spend much less time practising and often left the program idling on my desktop for days on end. There was one saving grace however, if I did get bored with my internet pursuits I would certainly pick up my virtual paintbrush and splash some oils around. It can be so much fun making up spontaneous images and rewarding if something special materializes.

On a cold January evening Emma finally gave birth to a son after being one week overdue. He was immediately named Iwan; it was one of the boys names Emma and Ceri had chosen a few weeks earlier. My parents along with Sian and myself were alerted to the wonderful news at about eight. We were all hyped up and buzzed about the news and wanted to tell the whole world! My mother was desperate to see Emma and her newborn son; quickly my father drove over to the hospital. Sian was left with me and we were given express instructions to tell as many friends and family members as we could.

Sian manned the phone and quickly called Uncle Alan, Aunty Rose and Uncle Don and our grandparents Beatrice and Henry. While Sian was excitedly telling our immediate family I was quietly tapping away on my mouse. Typing emails to my friends and to my mothers' friend Sue who lives in England. I lost track of all the people I'd told and was happily smiling away like the Cheshire cat from Alice in wonderland. I couldn't wait for my mother to get home so we could see the first beautiful pictures of my newborn nephew. By the time nine thirty arrived, Sian and I were all chatted out and waited with suspense for my parents to return.

As ten o'clock neared my parents walked through the front door quite clearly overjoyed. My mother was beaming and my father was busily telling us all that had happened after the birth. I asked about Emma and Ceri, finding out that mother and baby were doing very well and that Ceri had been great all the way through. My mother put a digital camera in front of me and was happily flicking through the picture list. "Aw he is so cute and tiny, did you have a hold Mam?" I said pleasantly. "Of course I did love, Nana had a hold" she said brightly. My mother then proceeded to show me the photograph of her holding Iwan. He weighed in at about seven pounds two ounces and looked adorable. We couldn't have been any prouder of Emma and Ceri; they were starting their very own family.

A few weeks later we got to see the latest addition to the family. Emma came in holding Iwan all wrapped up in a shawl; tucked up in a way that held him close. She of course was beaming from ear to ear but also looked extremely tired; the birth must have been exhausting. I'll never know how that one feels, being a guy and everything! "Em, Can I hold Alf....I mean Iwan" I said in embarrassment. I always had trouble remembering Iwan as he had been Alfie for nine months. Eventually I came around to saying his name correctly and that certainly saved my blushes. Emma agreed to let me hold him and gently approached my wheelchair; Iwan was all bundled up and unaware as he slept.

He felt so light and his blankets were warm against my awkward and unmoving arms. I was in awe as I'd never held a baby before. He smelt of *Johnsons' baby oil* and that almost imperceptible newborn smell. He was adorably sweet and gently murmured in his sleep. As I was quietly talking to him, saying how special and brilliant he was, he opened his small eyes for just a few seconds. At that precise moment my mother took a photo of me looking straight into his eyes. I could have held him there all night transfixed on this tiny bundle gently sleeping in my arms. Soon enough though the rest of my family began to hold him and tell him stories about the brave new world he had entered. It was a magical way to bring in the New Year and we all love him beyond measure.

I got back into the online pool league a bit more in February and really started to 'live' in the room. Demi and I would say we were part of the furniture. Most people thought I was great and a good friend, even though sometimes they would joke about me being a censor. It was all part of the charm of being a tournament director and I revelled in it. The sense of camaraderie between the staff was really high and there was always a contest to see who could host the most. One evening after I had hosted six tournaments back to back, Demi's partner told me that all the Admins were very pleased with my commitment. Great things would come if I kept at it and that gave me a boost and an impetus to carry on performing.

The league was so popular that getting members to join in was fairly easy; often we had up to twenty or thirty people in every evening. That is considered quite large by league standards. There were over two hundred active players (regularly attending members). You could see lots of different faces and I knew a lot of their names off by heart. I indeed felt like part of the furniture, maybe something French polished from the Edwardian era! It is amazing what you witness in these rooms; one minute there's a huge joke being spread around with the odd innuendo thrown in too (not too much as it was a family room); the next minute there's huge argument that needs to be dealt with. I'm either a teacher, a friend or I'm mediating between Eight ball disputes.

It's so fast and frenetic in there that I would often be staring at the screen with my mouth slightly open 'catching flies'. My mother often had to ask me a question three or more times before I finally registered it. At the height of my abilities; I could host two tournaments together, talk to people on the messenger and play pool. Thank goodness I had a light mouse otherwise that would have been impossible! By the end of the day my arms would ache and my mind felt totally numb; it was hard but rewarding work pleasing the masses. I slept really well after my hectic days and felt like I'd finally given something back to the world.

The reward for my hard work was a promotion to the position of head tournament director. I was so excited to be trusted this much and I really wanted to impress everyone. The new duties I was expected to do were more behind the scenes and staff related. All HTD's had a certain number of TD's below them and we were there to make sure they kept up their duties. If we found anyone who hadn't hosted in a few weeks, we were to send late letters and gentle reminders. If people were generally busy with other commitments then we would be lenient or put them on vacation. Vacation was a total break from TD'ing and playing in the league for an amount of days agreed by the Admin and TD in question. It was all fairly simple really.

Back in the room my workload increased with a lot more query answering and general tournament hosting. My *Yahoo* messenger was like a red hot emergency phone and increasingly I had less time to play pool myself. I learnt to deal with only the most important messages and not feel bad about passing problems on. During my time as HTD I taught many new TD's the ropes and my charges did very well and appreciated my help. I was always asking if they understood my given instructions and if not I was patient and guiding. I only hope they still enjoy being TD's and maybe even some of them are training the future recruits as I write this. Just as I thought my life couldn't get any fuller or exciting, it did! Well at least I thought it did as you will soon read.

It was a normal day sitting in front of my computer as the sun gently caressed the house in all its brilliant glory. The chat bar was full with the scrolling text of jokes and the odd argument too. I tapped away warning the two arguers to bear in mind that this was a family room and we need to keep it clean and fair. After a few more argumental moments the room settled down into its usual light-hearted banter. I turned my music player on and enjoyed some trance music I'd recently purchased. I believe it was called *Tranceport* by *Paul Oakenfold*, it was a compilation CD that I'd found on *Amazon*. I was listening to my favourite song at the time *Rendezvous [Quadraphonic Mix]* by *Tilt*.

As the song was reaching its first crescendo a message box popped up on my screen. It was a now defunct private message facility that was in every pool room. It was from one of the members I'd seen hanging around for a few weeks. Her ID was a curious letter and number combination that made me smile. She was figuring me out I guess, she was friendly and seemed cool but at the same time slightly cheeky. For a few days she kept messaging me after which I'd ascertained she was from a distant far eastern country and she knew I was from Wales. She didn't know where it was at first but after a few *Google* maps she kind of understood. She spent quite a lot of time talking to me and I loved the company. All the attention made me feel really special and needed. Most members just kept the conversation short expecting you to provide entertainment but this was so much more.

Every time we entered the room fresh from a break we greeted each other with huge virtual hugs. I always looked forward to that small bit of affection. My disease has taken away so much from me, including the ability to hug someone just for the heck of it. You kind of feel isolated and trapped within your own body even when you want to do something. By now if we wanted to talk we would set up a private pool table and play some games. I usually kept the table on screen while I did my work. We continued chatting to each other about our respective countries and asked about family and friends, it was so good talking things over with a person who cared for me. I told her about my disease and she didn't seem shocked or particularly bothered by it. She was in training to be a nurse so I suppose she read a lot about diseases.

I was pleased and relaxed that I'd broken the ice about being severely ill without any major dramas. We never seemed to argue and whenever she was sad it made me feel terrible. I would busily try to cheer her up and say something funny as I don't like to see anyone upset or sad. She responded with gentleness and affection and I was really happy that I could please someone else even though we were thousands of miles apart. We were getting 'close' all of a sudden and I remember telling my mother about this special girl I'd found. My mother didn't say much but I'm sure she was pleased that I was happy and contented.

One night at the start of June my new close friend said the words I thought I would never hear again in my life. She tapped out something along the lines of "Ian hunni, I love you so much and I want to be with you <3". I was totally blown away by this admission. I thought many quick thoughts; was this the love I was looking for; did I really feel the same way and what about the distance. I certainly cared greatly for her and I definitely could feel a certain kind of longing to be with her too. She was all I could think of and all I ever dreamed about. This must be love I thought! I tapped my response out "...I love you too and I would love it if you were with me! Big cuddles..." We then spent the next hour trying to say good bye as we were tired and sleepy. It was hard finally switching off the messenger we must have virtually hugged and kissed each other hundreds of times.

I know some people would think it silly of me to hug someone 'virtually' but it was all I had and I clung on to hope. I had many wonderful dreams of meeting her off a plane and showing her all of Wales and finally feeling her embrace. I would have given up a million virtual hugs for just one slow meaningful kiss but I just couldn't allow myself to think that far ahead. I discussed these things with Miss B (as I will refer to her from now on) during a lull in the pool room. I finally asked "How long until we could meet in person..." I nervously typed. She responded "...well hunni, I've got two or three years left of studies, I could see you maybe then..." So could I wait until then I mulled over in my mind. I thought I'm sure I can still be here in three years and was determined to make it. I could feel the passion building up in me; I was willing DMD not to take me yet!

Once that sticky issue was dealt with, we had a fairly uneventful month. Our bond seemed to grow deeper and deeper over the bright days and warm nights. I heard her voice the first time over the messenger, what a truly marvellous invention the internet is! Her voice sounded so much older than her nineteen years but it was still charming and young. I heard her cool accent which sounded far eastern but with the hint of an American brogue. I was worried that we wouldn't be able to understand each other but very quickly we stumbled through to an understanding. It was so fulfilling to hear her saying my name and she loved the way I said hers. I could have talked for hours but it was late there she had to go so as not to wake her family. We said our tender good nights and painfully I shut everything down.

Just as everything was finally settling down in my personal life, issues started to arise in my voluntary work life. It was the start of a very painful week. One morning I awoke to find that all the Admins had decided to up and leave, without telling me before hand. I was in shock and terribly upset that my friends had all left me to it. The reason behind it all was the return of the leagues rightful Head Admin. She had been very abrupt, condescending and generally horrid to Demi and company. Of course Demi told me how upset this made her but she never really explicitly laid down what had been going on. I can see now why they had to leave but back then I felt abandoned and wondered what would happen to the team now.

I had never really spoken to this Head Admin and didn't know of her true personality. From the meetings I had with her in the room and on the messenger, I found her pleasant, friendly and generally positive. I was in the middle between my friends and this person I hardly knew. If I knew and truly felt she was abusive I would have left in heartbeat but she fooled me into believing she was kind and welcoming. I decided to stay and see for myself what it was like to work with this new HA. Demi seemed to never acknowledge the fact that at the time I didn't have any quarrel with the HA. We had many painful arguments about this and it made me feel unwell. I felt I had been made to feel like a pariah for staying put.

The league felt like my home I had loads of friends still in there. I just felt torn three ways, torn by my friends, my league and this unknown quantity of an HA. The next day I was offered a promotion to be an Admin as obviously the league had just lost three the day before. I had wanted to be an Admin for about two months before this fateful day. I could see the league needing an extra pair of administrative hands and I thought this may be my only chance before my hands weakened or even worse. I jumped at the offer thinking all my dreams would be answered. Demi however thought I was snubbing her and our friends and I felt truly awful; why was this dividing our friendship!

Over the course of the next five days my workload exploded as the new HA pushed more and more things in my direction. After my training I now had to deal with hundreds of queries, member and staff disputes, check the leagues emails, check the activity logs, monitor potential fraudulent accounts and host tournaments. I was drowning under all the work but I never once complained and Miss B was a star helping me to relax. It was hard work but our love seemed just as strong even after the upheaval with our friends. Meanwhile the HA was nowhere to be seen, some evenings she would check in and give me even more work. To add insult she would constantly tell me how awful Demi was. I knew full well that Demi was a kind, hardworking and dedicated person so it cut into my heart every time.

I told Demi all the lies the HA was saying and my plight with the overload of work. I got upset and nearly cried as we discussed everything but Demi was very comforting and tried to help me figure out my work issues. Our friendship wasn't dead after all! I felt so relieved that we weren't enemies I had always respected Demi; we were virtual mother and son. She said something about her joining another league but I didn't take it in as I was still stressed. By day six I was at my wits end, I'd only played two or three games of pool in that week and all of the work started to affect my health.

I had been feeling constantly sick, I just couldn't eat at all; the smell of food was making me heave. I was always stressed, panicky and very down. On the seventh day I had to step down from my position with immediate affect. My body had decided enough was enough; I simply couldn't ignore it any longer. I explained to the HA how much I wasn't coping, she was at first disappointed but said she 'understood'. I felt so much better out of the vice like grip of stress and constant angst. In no time I felt well enough to eat again and my mood lifted considerably. Being out of the TD loop felt liberating, I could now be with my girl a lot more and play pool which had become a real luxury lately.

One late night after Miss B had safely gone to sleep I felt like exploring the other pool rooms in the *Yahoo* universe. Remembering vaguely that Demi had joined a new league I decided to try and find her and our friends. Demi couldn't tell me the league's name or it's location due to general league rules. She never revealed anything to me as Demi is an honourable, rule abiding person. So instead I had to trawl every room to see if I recognised any of my friends. I spent about two hours looking until finally I stumbled upon a quiet room with very few passing visitors. Demi was sat there in an old ID I barely remembered along with our other friends. It felt like the prodigal son had returned and I was welcomed with wide open arms; the old gang were back together!

Very quickly I learned that Demi and her partner had started a brand new league just a few weeks prior. I had no idea they were even planning to start another league. I was so overjoyed to have found them that the next night I signed up. It was so exciting to be starting out after the birth of a new league and I couldn't wait to show Miss B. You are allowed to be in two leagues at the same time as long as you don't work for them i.e. as a TD. Obviously I had just quit working for my original league due to health issues so I was fine in that respect. All progressed well for the next few days that is until the HA of my first league found out!

Incandescent with rage the HA finally showed her true colours. It was the one of most frightening outbursts I'd seen on my messenger. She sent wild accusations in my direction, she thought Demi had put me up to this and somehow Demi must have told me to step down. I held my ground by telling the truth, "I went and joined Demi's league off my own back, it was my decision and I quit Admin due to stress and sickness". She was having none of it and kept attacking me, finally saying "obviously you faked your illness as an excuse to cover your butt". I was shocked, hurt and saddened by the fact that she called me a liar. I simply don't lie about my health as I have no need too; it is something I'd never think of doing! Outraged by this badgering and all of her twisted lies I decided to leave my first league and never return. I was sad it all ended badly after my dedication but I have forgiven her even if she still thinks ill of me.

# The Lift Debacle

My personal problems all seemed to be levelling out around me but as I know only too well life tends to throw a spanner in the works. That spanner in this case was my old grey lift. It had been my loyal servant for a shade over a decade, but time and wear had started to take its toll. For the last six months a rather alarming intermittent fault kept occurring often at the most annoying times. While going down between floors the loudest of crushing reverberating bangs would emanate above my head. My heart would pound as I was trapped in a metal box stopped and suspended ten feet above the floor. I didn't know what had caused this stoppage but at the time I didn't care; all I wanted was out of there!

My mother hearing all this commotion came rushing over to see if I was alright. After establishing that I was ok but a bit shaken up she quickly called the council's lift repair engineer. He was in the area and fortunately popped in to see if he could help. After a few minutes in deep thought he looked all around the lift from above and below and told me it's either a problem with the chain or possibly the limit switches. As this was a lift he was unfamiliar with and quite old by the councils' standards he didn't really know what to do. Twenty minutes later my father returned home from work to discover my predicament; he then attempted to correct the problem.

He stood on top of the lift trying to solve the problem; being a mechanical engineer really helps in these kinds of situations. A few minutes passed by and he finally started to correct the chain by physically moving it. There were a number of limit switches surrounding the chain; if one of these was activated by any stray movement then the lift would be stopped. My father straightened the chain, got off the top of the lift and pressed the lower button; immediately the lift roared into life and started to move. The tired but loud motor inched me down and thirty seconds later I landed on the ground floor totally relieved. I couldn't wait to get out, the anxiety made me tired and jumpy. I needed to relax and cool down in front of my gently whirring laptop.

For the next few months this kept happening but luckily my father was always around. One memorable occasion at around one in the morning; I got into my lift on the ground floor ready for bed; when again the reverberating clatter sounded! I thought "Oh great, I want to go to bed! Why has this got to happen now?" I grunted in sheer desperation as I sat in my lift. Quickly my mother had to run upstairs to wake my father. The poor guy was half asleep, with his eyes barely open he asked "What's up?" I then told him "It's the same loud bang... the chain must have slipped again!" Gingerly my father lowered himself down the lift shaft from my bedroom via a long ladder. By the time he was on top of the lift he came around and immediately corrected the chain. We all drifted off to sleep that night annoyed at the lift and its impromptu stoppages.

The final straw however was on a barmy June afternoon just after I finished playing pool. After telling Miss B that I needed a break for a few minutes; I rung my mother from the family computer and asked "Mam, Can I come down?" I often used *Skype* to call my mother because my voice was getting considerably weaker. So after the quick phone call; my mother helped me in to the lift and pressed the lower button. About three feet down the almighty bang resounded yet again, I was frightened and my heart was pounding away. I then had a sickening realisation that my father was at least an hour and a half away from getting home! My mother knew that the council's lift repair man wouldn't know what to do but she had to do something.

Forty minutes later the guy turned up and made his way to where I was suspended. He bumbled about checking the chain and talking to me all the while scratching his head. He really didn't have a clue and was assuring me that the lift should be condemned. Not that it was necessarily faulty but because it was too old and unfamiliar to the repairmen. When he stated "...oh we might have to cut the chain...I think..." I really started to panic! "Won't I fall?" I gasped out. "No you'll be ok buddy!" he said to me confidently. I thought a little too confident for my liking. The next hour dragged on painfully as the man rang various colleagues back at base and poked around the chain.

I told him that he should try to straighten the chain but it just fell on deaf ears. Just as I thought I would be spending the night in a draughty metal box my father came home! I was giddy and giggling with relief as I thought "...it won't be long now till I'm free!" My father put his briefcase away then came up to my lift and in next to no time he had righted the chain. It seemed my father was the only one who could sort my lift out; that must have put a terrible pressure upon him, although he didn't show it. He was my hero for getting me free so many times. After my two hour ordeal I was cold, tired and hugely annoyed. "We have got to get a new lift! After that thing trapped me again..." I said passionately. Happily my parents' agreed with me.

In the space of about three weeks we had builders come in to size up the task of replacing my old lift for a newer model. The chief builder was a tall man with a bushy moustache who always had plenty of jokes. He was very quick to come up with a plan of action and would proceed almost immediately. The night before they were due to come in my father decided to start work ready by dismantling a non vital part of the lift. I was up in my room already, for the next few days I was told I would be spending the duration in my bedroom while the lift was being replaced.

The next day the work commenced with loud banging and singing builders! I was moved in to my mother's bedroom, which took an awful lot of manoeuvring and shoving of my wheelchair. I was wedged in next my mother's bed playing on my laptop. The builders had told my father off for starting work ahead of time, but you can't stop a curious engineer I thought! My mother came back and forth checking on me as I sitting next to a sunny window. It was nearly oppressive in my mothers' room but fortunately a cool breeze was wafting through the room via a fan. It was quite difficult to see my screen as the sun poured though the thin curtains but I was comfortable and busy playing pool.

Every night the builders would take off at about five in the afternoon and I would squeeze my way out of my parent's room. Just avoiding the top of the stairs I swung my chair skilfully back into my bedroom. It was like opening a tin of sardines! I was tired sweaty and hungry after spending six hours wedged next to a bed in the hot sunshine. Thankfully my bedroom was like a cool oasis and soon enough I was watching the wall mounted TV whilst tapping away on the family PC. My father had moved the PC along with its large metal desk into the front room of my bedroom. There was just enough space for me, the bed and the PC with a certain amount of manoeuvring but I was fairly content.

My temporary accommodation was basic now that I couldn't get downstairs, but I was assured that within seven days my new lift would be ready. I had no access to the bath or the toilet so I was left with an ugly chemical commode for company. I would keep using the computer till about ten thirty talking over everything with Miss B, but she couldn't really understand my situation. When ten thirty arrived I had to try to go to the toilet, it was my usual time to go. My mother hooked me up via my grey sling onto the hoist and up I went dangling above my bed. Next she would move my wheelchair away and replace it with the ugly plastic and steel commode. Then I'm lowered onto it. It was very uncomfortable, poking my thighs and stinging my back. I couldn't get into correct position so unsurprisingly I couldn't go!

Getting into bed my stomach was growling in protest after the failed attempt to relieve myself. I feel asleep counting down the hours, minutes and seconds until I could see downstairs again! The back room was in a shambles, the lift shaft was taken out leaving a gapping hole in the floor and parts of the ceiling were loose. They dismantled the lift in an hour which surprised me, because as a child it felt like it took an age to build. It was strange to see how much larger the back room was now that the shaft was removed. The 'shaft' in fact was made up of two small partition walls but for all the years we had it I never seemed to put two and two together. In my mind I had imagined it was made of steel not the flimsy wood it turned out to be.

The next seven days dragged by slowly as the builders finished preparing the hole and sorting out the floor. Curiously we had heard very little from the company making my lift but no one seemed too concerned. Towards the end of the week the builders had less and less to do; eventually just left to sweeping up the floor. I thought in a few days time I would finally go downstairs and be able to properly use the facilities! The pain was becoming a little more intense as each day passed but I was tolerating it well. My mother had been plying me with laxatives but my bowels seemed immoveable, my body really hated using an uncomfortable commode.

Miss B had loads of advice because of her nursing course but still nothing seemed to work. I was glad however to give my love to my attractive girlfriend who was caring and affectionate right back at me.

The week ended in total despair and panic as we were told something awful. A council representative dealing with our lift renewal informed us that the lift company had pulled out. Apparently it was too difficult of a job for them so they gave up; leaving me literally high and dry! At first I was incredulous and confused thinking "How could it be too difficult?" My father was very angry at this pitiful display by a company we were assured were up to the task. My mother was extremely upset and often tempers would fray with every one of us snapping cross words. I felt terrible, a mixture of fear and anxiety was flashing through my mind and it was all I could do not to cry.

My father was definitely not letting the council off the hook and demanded they help us to find a new lift company as soon as possible. It took quite awhile to sift through potential companies and often at night my father would ring around checking on them. About two weeks later we finally spoke to a nice enough bloke called "Drew" from a lift company in South West England. He came over to our house to check out the work already completed. He wasn't entirely happy with what he saw; the new enlarged hole was way off centre. More work had to be completed before any new lift could be installed. It was quickly assured that this work would be done and later we learned that Drew's company was indeed going to install my new lift. The only issue being that it would take three months!

Horrified at this delay both my father and myself asked, "Is there any alternative to that!?" The only other thing Drew could suggest was the use of a smaller temporary hire lift. My father was very keen to go ahead and I could see a small ray of hope ahead of me. To see if I could fit into a temporary lift, Drew told us the measurements and my father mocked up an area of my room to the same dimensions. After various attempts trying to reverse into the space I finally cracked it immediately feeling the relief washing over me. There was one snag however it would take five weeks for it to arrive. That was considerably quicker than three months but it seemed inevitable I would have to become intimately acquainted with my bedroom!

The next five weeks dragged by like a prison sentence. I could see the sunny days but I couldn't get out there, downstairs could have been on Mars for all I knew. After much pain, pushing and exhaustion I managed to use the commode but it certainly wasn't what you'd call normal. I had grown used to the discomfort but I'd often grimace and hear my stomachs angry protestations. I kept it mostly to myself whilst talking to my friends, I'm sure some people never even knew I was having a crisis at home. Miss B was as understanding as she could be from the other side of the world but she kept me going with her presence. It would have been awful to do this alone. Every night we would continue our love filled routine of many virtual hugs, kisses and we would exchange virtual roses.

So that my mother didn't go insane we continued to have our fortnightly crossroads carers in. She and my father went out to bingo and I stayed with Rita and Carol watching my small TV. They were obviously concerned to see me left high and dry and asked all about what had happened. I was tired and really couldn't be bothered to give a full account so I quickly ran through the problems. Every day I would run through it in my mind getting increasingly agitated so I really didn't want to talk about it over and over. It was great to see friendly faces though. I had no visiting friends because most people I knew were in America or in other corners of the World. Demi was in London but that is a fair way from me, I couldn't expect her to drop everything to see me.

At last after a total of eight weeks stranded in my room the temporary lift arrived! I was overcome with excitement as I was finally released from my prison cell of a room. It was a tight squeeze getting in but after a few elbow scrapes and some wheel locking I was there. Coming downstairs seemed ridiculously easy after my enforced incarceration and I felt relieved to finally see the outside world. I sat in the garden for a good while lapping up the sweet smells and feeling a delightful breeze playing with my hair. I had a big smile plastered on my face for about three days and I finally used the facilities that I'd missed the most. I was very tired of struggling on that small ugly plastic bin they had the audacity to call a commode!

I still had a few weeks to wait for the proper lift as my twenty second birthday came and went by. In the meantime it was pretty much business as usual. My elbows were getting a beating from my lift entry exploits and a fair sized bruise had come up. It was all worth it though just to be free from my small front bedroom area. I really did feel like a released prisoner out on good behaviour! The tensions decreased greatly during the hire lift period; save for the cost of hiring the lift. It was left to my father to pay the few hundred pounds it cost for the privilege of using it. In my opinion the least the company that let us down could have done was to pay that fee but it wasn't to be.

Eventually the time passed and over a sunny weekend a few lift engineers replaced the temporary lift with my permanent model. Again I had to spend it back in my bedroom commuting ten feet across our narrow landing into my parents' room by day. I was at ease though because I knew the guys were working on it, by the first night it was almost complete. The lift ran up two metal boxed sections powered by a small piston located in the right stanchion from the lift users' perspective. The lift proper was yet to be installed and it consisted of a through floor plate which concealed the lift while it was downstairs and the open plan metal car. I was feeling quite excited that I was finally getting a brand new modern looking lift put in. It had been an awful long wait just getting to this point; we sorely wanted it over and done with. It's never ending the trouble Duchenne families go through just to get the most basic of services, but you have just got to keep fighting and maybe one day things will change.

I had so much fun trying out the new 'Harmony' lift that I must have rode up and down in it for ages. It was so liberating using that new machine but at first I had trouble getting my head around the new open plan feeling. I felt slightly dizzy having been used to a cramped temporary lift which scraped my arms. Now though I had plenty of elbow room and even space to take my suctioning machine. All of that made my mother and me very happy, it was one less worry upon our heads. My father was intrigued by the whole lift assembly procedure and asked many questions of the main engineer Paul. By five in the evening Paul and his crew had finished all their assembly and were bidding us good bye as the sunshine started to go hazy. At last I had my new lift!

# *Age Twenty-Two*

Around the time of my twenty second birthday when the temporary lift (mentioned in the last chapter) was installed. My life settled down almost back to normality, so I could at least spend more time with Miss B. By now we had been dating 'online' for approximately two months and everything seemed brilliant. We would spend lots of time talking at the pool tables or chatting on the messenger. Miss B seemed to care for me a lot and I was so besotted with her, I would do anything for that girl! I was so happy thinking I had found the 'one' so much so we were even discussing a possible future wedding with friends. Everyone in Demi's new league loved Miss B and I, Demi's partner would often comment "Ah young love!"

Unfortunately things started to fall apart and I stubbornly refused to see it until it was too late. I remember thinking at the time "What is happening to me?" I had changed and I wasn't proud of myself for it. Miss B would say snide vitriolic remarks about the other women that I was friends with. She put me under pressure not to 'virtually' hug or kiss my friends or to even talk to them. She had me believing all her jealousy and all her lies. I would often end up snapping at friends or having blazing arguments with others. I can remember accusing a friend of being horrible and threatening to Miss B; shamefully I believed her rubbish. After that I felt awful and guilt wracked, I could see I was turning into something I despised. The fear of losing someone close just kept me agreeing with Miss B.

After she had subdued me into being little more than a 'yes' man, she began to turn on me and I just let her get on with it. I never once questioned her. She pushed me so hard to produce tournament after tournament all for her selfish pleasure. I was becoming increasingly tired and it didn't seem to matter one bit to her. Some days were completely different as she would leave me on my own for hours with no explanations and come back full of irritability. I wasn't allowed to leave like that otherwise she would become hysterical. I had to tell her when I was eating and she'd make me leave the pool room until I had finished. Miss B kept twisting me in the wind and I would still profess my love to her! I would still tell my mother how much I loved Miss B, I even wanted to fly her over here but fortunately my father refused.

I say fortunately because three months into our relationship the most painful discussion happened. I asked Miss B if she wanted to "see a picture of me on my ventilator" and pleasingly she agreed. I had talked all about my disease and she knew I used a ventilator; she seemed to be at ease with this. I showed her a picture of me with my facemask on and my eyes softly looking out, she wanted to see the real me and a big part of that is my ventilator. Painfully she was horrified saying "I feel sick, I don't want to see that!" and "I'm not ready". I was very hurt and felt betrayed by the woman who was supposed to love me. I wondered how she could say that after three months and after all the intimate things we discussed. She was training to be a nurse too! When I talked about it to her she just shut me down moving on to other topics. I told her "I feel like an ugly monster" and she refused to even acknowledge my feelings.

Two weeks later in our fourth month I felt thoroughly awful and used. In a difficult decision I knew I had to make, it was time to leave her. It was hard because of all the great plans we had and all those dreams we shared. Also I didn't want to leave a relationship, would I ever find love again? I just couldn't get over the hurt she inflicted on me though and what I had become to my friends. I just didn't talk to them any longer and I missed the friendly banter. It was high time that I took responsibility and set the record straight with Miss B. I told her "I feel like a convenience store boyfriend, you pick and choose when you want me!" She was dumfounded and when I said it's over she put the tears on and sent a lot of guilt my way. I just switched the computer off. I still felt upset and numb though as my mother walked in.

I had so many mixed emotions I just broke down in tears. My mother gave me a hug and reassured me that it was the right thing to do. I was crying at the loss of a relationship and the pain of the "sick" comment and for hurting my friends. I took most of the day to recover but began to feel better again the next day. Sadly and embarrassingly I went back to Miss B after a relentless guilt trip as she promised change. At the end of a week however I saw nothing but the same old behaviour.

I finally broke off contact on a quiet Sunday afternoon, I severed all ties, deleting her off messenger and ignoring her emails. For the coming next year I would hate her and try to get her removed from Demi's league. I was so angry and hurt that I couldn't let it go not until very recently at least. Now I've forgiven her completely and it makes life a whole lot easier just to move on and forget.

The few weeks after Miss B were the hardest to cope with, I was hurting and I felt completely lost. My routine of talking to someone everyday was shattered and loneliness set in really quickly. Each day felt boring and I still felt numb after all that had gone on before. Then something marvellous happened, one of my friends whom I thought I'd hurt, consoled me and was really sweet and caring towards me. Everyday she would make me laugh and virtually hug me loads of times. She would laugh at my strange Welsh words and she started to show me some Spanish words she had learnt in high school. We had known each other about a year and she was and still is a good friend. She lives in America and spoke with a beautiful northern states accent.

She told me all about Miss B; she knew what she was like as they had been friends in a different league for awhile. You may wonder why didn't she warn me, but at the time she did say and she did warn me however I was too stubborn and obsessed with Miss B. I didn't want to listen as I tend to just see the good in people but not the bad; possibly I'm a little naïve in that department. This sweet loving American girl seemed so much different from Miss B she was a complete antithesis in fact. This new young woman also revealed something she had kept hidden from me for a few months. She told me she was starting to fall in love with me but before she could tell me, Miss B came in and claimed me as her phony prize.

The next week we started talk more deeply and more intimately and I could see she was genuine and truly did care for me. It was no act like that of my previous fraught relationship. I felt a connection with this woman that I couldn't quite define. She made me feel special, loved, useful and human again not like the machine Miss B wanted. I hope I made her feel the same way about me after all I thought I would never find love again. Then not even three weeks later I found what seemed like the girl of my dreams, she didn't care that I was paralysed and living with DMD. Miss C (as I'll now refer to her due to confidentiality) just saw the person and not the disease and my picture didn't sicken her!

Some may think this was a "rebound" but I had to give love a try. How many opportunities did I have left? After all she said she loved me and it just felt right to me in my heart. Something inside me told me to go for it; surely this *must* be what real love is. I could feel myself falling in love, it wasn't the constant messaging of Miss B; this was a mutual attraction of minds. I finally talked about my feelings with her and tentatively asked if I could be her boyfriend. I was so nervous typing all of that to her but wonderfully she said something along the lines of "...Of course you can be my boyfriend! ..." I was feeling extremely pleased and wonderful. She was so sweet and interested in me that I thought this was so going to work!

The first couple of weeks with Miss C were fantastic and I can only sum it up as pure bliss. I could say what I wanted to anyone and it was great to be finally trusted. I had no problem trusting Miss C as we had known each other awhile and she was wonderfully up front and determined. We talked about everything from our favourite pool game right up to serious issues surrounding my disease. She said something sweet about the distance we were apart that I often remember, "If we never see each other, at least we'll meet in heaven". I was touched by the sincerity and tenderness Miss C showed toward me and I struggled to answer her. It was a fantastic faith that despite all our troubles there could be more; but at the same time it felt bittersweet.

I knew realistically I hadn't got that long left before my disease killed me and took me away from everyone I knew and loved. I don't know precisely when that fateful day will occur but every year I get worse; I lose something more and get increasingly isolated. Transatlantic flights are a dream to me it was just too far of a journey and I couldn't face the hassles and discomforts that would arise. Just sitting on a plane brings with it a nine hour wait in a chair not designed for pressure relief. I could land in excruciating pain just travelling to see someone I loved. All of this led me to ask when Miss C could possibly come visit me, she said "...it could possibly be 6 years before I could visit Europe..."

At first I just said "Oh right" but it began to play on my mind night and day. I would lay awake thinking that I maybe couldn't last six years. I couldn't talk it over with Miss C because I didn't know how I could broach the subject. I was nervous that she would take it the wrong way; I knew she couldn't leave America for all that time and I knew I couldn't leave Wales. I was also extremely concerned by what my condition would be like in that future time. Would I be dead or would I be in state of high distress; I just couldn't land that on Miss C. She would have qualifications and want a career; I couldn't imagine her throwing it all away for me. I know she was willing to do that but I just didn't feel it would work out. I didn't want to be selfish and make her leave everything.

One morning I discussed this with my mother and told her that I was going to have to end my relationship with Miss C. I was so nervous and unsure about the future because I knew being twenty two with DMD you certainly can't bank on at least six years. It was so upsetting to think that this couldn't really work; the distance between us and my uncertain future were too great an obstacle. When I saw Miss C later on during a now cold September evening I just couldn't do it. I couldn't break her heart! My current condition and future deterioration were like two sniper rifles pointing at my head. I couldn't ignore it and hope all things Duchenne would go away. It took me a further three days to pluck up the courage to drive a nail through another relationship.

Depressingly I bit the bullet so to speak and initiated a conversation that I still have mixed feelings about today. Miss C came on the messenger her usual bright, funny and determined self. I just came out with something like, "...hun, I don't think this is going to work; we're going to have to end our relationship..." I was immediately gutted but I had to go through with it. Miss C, bless her heart thought my account had been hacked by an imposter, she said, "...this isn't Ian! It's totally not like him..." To prove it was me she started a voice conversation between us and had me talk. Terribly sad I quickly proved it was me and Miss C understandably became upset. We continued our conversation on the messenger when she asked something like "...Ok, but why must you end things?"

I then told her about the distance between us and how difficult it would be for me to wait six years or possibly more. We then argued for a good few hours trying to convince each other that this either was or wasn't going to work out. In the end Miss C reluctantly came to a similar conclusion to me but I'm not sure she ever really agreed. I was exhausted and felt totally hollow; it was the second time I had to end a relationship and become the 'enemy' again. Immediately after those tortuous moments, we went our separate ways and didn't really talk any further that night. As I slept later things began flowing through my mind and deep regrets bubbled to the surface; did I really want this? I agonized over this decision but still my heart felt deeply attached to her.

About two days later after thinking constantly I'd made the biggest mistake of my life; I wanted to ask Miss C if she'd take me back. Firstly when I saw her I was glad we were still talking and I gently broached the subject of getting back together. I don't know weather I was sad or relieved by her response. In her determined way she said "...well I agree with you, it would never work out, we live too far apart..." I felt mixed emotions at the time

I felt the loss of another companion and I knew this was the permanent end to things. Being just friends after that point was very hard and I was confused not knowing whether I was virtually hugging her too much or saying inappropriate things. Well we are still good friends now but it has taken me so long to truly move on and she still holds a special place in my heart. Sometimes "If only things were different" enters my mind whenever I reminisce about Miss C.

Towards the end of September and by the beginning of October no-one online really talked to me. There were no women to console me this time. For the first time in five long months I had many moments to think; that's when everything hit me. Two failed relationships and being stranded in my bedroom were too much for my mind to take. Depression washed over my body filling my mind with all sorts of desperate thoughts. This disease robbing me of relationships and slowly eating my muscles made me upset. I was truly desperately missing tender conversations and being loved by another. My other friends couldn't say anything to cheer me up; all I could think was "What's the point of going on?"

I couldn't feel any happiness; my moods were like the weather outside, dark and oppressively foreboding. I was quiet at home and constantly thought about how awful I felt. Unlike me there were no smiles, very few jokes and a general malaise. Why couldn't I find the woman I so wanted and needed? Why did this disease have to keep snatching things away from me? All these negative things collided in my brain, like flak hitting a flying fortress, constant and painful. I kept thinking I had made big mistakes all through my life and should I be stronger than this? I had gone with the flow all along but now I felt unable to go on; stuck in a rut of bad feelings running on an everlasting loop. Some dark nights I even mulled over suicide but something just told me to pull away from that idea.

After finally telling my mother I was feeling so unusually low she tried to get me to see all the positives in my life. My wonderful nephew and my great family and all I had done in online Eight ball pool. It just didn't work for me; I felt like nothing could lift me out of this pit of hopelessness. Another evening my mother told me that perhaps I should ask my doctor about anti-depressants. That just sent my mind into frenzy, on the one hand I could see it working but on the other I thought I don't want to take that kind of medication. Another complication was that the doctor I see was a regular respiratory consultant, I felt really uncomfortable talking to a guy who doesn't deal with the mind. The thought of talking it over with him daunted me as I tend to mumble or get quite shy; I decided there must be another way!

Firstly I tried music to lift my spirits out of the lowness I was feeling. In the beginning it was hopeless; a slightly slower tune would set me off crying. Strangely I kept going back to these sad songs almost as if I needed them. I would sit upstairs in my bedroom fighting back tears and choking up; I was trying to keep the noise down so as not to alert my mother. I just had to let it out, tell myself things were unfair and listen to the sad songs I was drawn too. *Far Away* by *Nickelback* is a tune that still makes me feel sad even when I occasionally listen to it now. Eventually I got tired of getting upset and crying that I focused on more positive songs. Rock songs really helped, I played all my *Stereophonics* songs into the ground! I love *Pick a part that's new* and *Step on my ol' size nines* and most of their older stuff.

Feeling slightly more like my old self after all that 'music' therapy albeit still quite sad. I needed to do something else to cheer me up; to let the happiness back into my life like a ray of sunshine. Remembering that I still had *Corel Painter IX* sitting on my laptop, I decided to fire it up and put all my feelings down in paint. The first images were just abstract sloshes of oil paint smeared on a white background. It was quite liberating forgetting about all my problems and about the sadness hanging over me like the dagger of Damocles. I began to work on an artwork project that I'd chip away at everyday; colouring and drawing small parts of an empty canvas. It was of two figures hugging each other surrounded by mist and car lights streaking away behind them. I called it *Freezing Arms* after a lyric on a *Snow Patrol* track.

At last I began to feel my depression lifting, I looked forward to my food and my smile came back. I felt renewed and determined after my inner turmoil settled. I wanted my positivity back and I wanted to fight my DMD to not let it consume my thoughts; I had got through life by not dwelling on things. Being creative and singing along to upbeat music was the torch of distraction I needed. Ideas started to flow in my mind like the crashing of ocean waves. Every dream I had brought forth these artistic ideas but I was unhappy with the quality of art I was producing. I kept at and practised more getting totally into the flow of things and before I knew it I was back to my old self! What a battle it had been over the period of a month, although I was now happier the dark thoughts are never too far away. Most people don't see it because I hide it convincingly under my positive attitude but it's a constant battle in the deep recesses of my mind.

October and November heralded a positive change in my life that I didn't expect. During one lonely evening hosting several tournaments in Demi's league I was chatting to one of the familiar faces; while we hadn't always got along, that evening marked somewhat of a truce. We were talking about the few pieces of art that I had made over the past weeks. He was very complementary about my pieces as were a few other people I had made gifts for. Suddenly out of the blue he mentioned a poet friend of his that displayed her work on an art website. The site was called *DeviantArt*, I was immediately intrigued. Unsure I asked what exactly did the site offer and my friend said it was a place where a community of all sorts of artists display their works and comment on them.

It would have been bold to call myself an 'artist' back then; I was firmly in the amateur category! I thought "what the heck" lets just check this site out and see if I'm compatible. The day after the conversation with my pool buddy I typed in *DeviantArt* on *Google* and hit 'search' with my mouse. There were tons of hits but you could tell which one was the art site. Shining out in blue the link I wanted said this; "deviantART: where ART meets application". What an exciting sounding heading I thought, it was bold and eye catching. I clicked the link and was transported to a greenish-grey website that certainly looked 'deviant' from the norm. I was confronted by works of art that just blew my mind with their sharp crisp professional images. I didn't think I stood a chance compared to these artists!

On further inspection I found far ranging pieces of art produced by teenager's right up to professional octogenarians. That gave me much more confidence so I thought lets check out the sign up procedure. I clicked a few buttons and was about to join when I was confronted with a huge list of terms and conditions. There were many admonishments about not stealing someone else's work and making sure everything was above board and beyond reproach. I was so new to art that I was daunted and felt totally lost, I'm such a worrier that I virtually ran a mile screaming! Frightened off fearing my work was not up to scratch I closed the *Deviantart* site and forgot about it. Instead I went back to hosting pool tournaments.

As if my friend was psychic he came into the pool room one day with his poet friend. She was an interesting girl with curious witty sometimes dark poetry skills. We got talking and I told her all about my fears with *Deviantart's* scary terms and conditions. She seemed pretty unconcerned telling me that *Deviantart* was a pretty laid back place as long as you produced your own work and respected copyright etc. Well I knew my work was/is original and I would always try to respect fellow artists. She put my mind right at ease and I quickly decided to sign up and give it a go. The poet became my first friend on *Deviantart* but sadly I don't see her much these days.

On my first full day as a member of the *Deviantart* community I did a heck of a lot of exploring. I saw beautiful photographs of gorgeous scenery right up to bizarre fractal images that throw your mind into chaos. I loved all the different genres of art and was always wondering, "Could I do that?" Any images you really like can be set as your 'favourites'; a small section on your user page is dedicated to displaying them. Every time you fancy dipping into the truly outstanding artworks you've seen on your travels through *DA* you can easily reach them. It's like a selection box of all the best chocolates you've had in you're life right at your finger tips. I am always blown away by the skills on show; they are truly inspirational because the images make you want to improve.

I decided to produce a new painting as my first ever 'deviation' (the term for an uploaded piece of art). Slowly I opened *Painter IX* and decided to use the palette knife tool to scrape away at some colourful oils. As quick as I could with my weakened hands I managed to scrape out a simple image of a beach. I wasn't overly impressed with what I'd created but it certainly wasn't awful. As my first piece for *Deviantart* it was definitely suitable and something to improve from. I uploaded it sometime in the afternoon not really expecting a huge response. A few hours later I checked back on my work to discover an awesome and wholly uplifting comment. It went something like this "...very simple but very effective...Your style is amazing, keep improving." There was also some advice on how to improve my next piece. It was a great first comment and I'm still hooked on *Deviantart* today.

I carried on adding more works over the next few months well into 2007. I experimented with different styles including abstract, surreal and my basic interpretation of realism. I painted anything from beaches at sunset to Demi's pet dog and even my favourite and ever ubiquitous drink *Pepsi Max*. I've always got one settling on my wheelchair table ready for a slurp! This new site really does develop your sense of community; it doesn't matter what problems you have because mostly anyone can produce something artistic. Over time I've made a few friendships and have seen some outstanding pieces of art. Hopefully as long as I'm able too, I'll still remain part of the *Deviantart* family.

# *Age Twenty-Three*

I can remember a very strong desire to get a webcam after I saw a section on *Deviantart* devoted to them. A few of my pool friends had let me see them on their cams so I thought why not give it go. *YouTube* was starting to become a worldwide phenomenon; I had seen a few other guys my age also living with DMD producing videos. I thought if these guys from America can do a video then why can't I? I kept suggesting to my mother that I wanted a webcam for my birthday, so she gave me permission to order one. I then trawled *Amazon* looking for a webcam that would suit me. I needed something small that could be operated via computer mouse as I can't physically move my arm to a camera. I was so excited waiting for the cam to arrive; I'd not been this excited for a good few years!

It arrived in the post on a particularly grey and humid July afternoon and soon after I opened it. I say open it but what I mean is getting my mother to do all the physical stuff; if I wasn't disabled I'd feel like a king! Although I would rather be able to do things myself, but I just take whatever life throws at me however painful. The week of my birthday turned out fiercely sunny which was a welcome change from the muggy weather we'd been having. In the end I picked a *Logitech* webcam that would fit above my laptop and on the family PC monitor (this allowed me some privacy). I could always get a few hours to myself whilst tapping away in my blue walled bedroom.

After a few days playing around with the settings and producing a few boring "Hi how are you?" testing videos I was ready for my first DMD related video. I wanted to tell people what I was going through with my disease and what caused the condition, with my usual positivity thrown in too. I wanted it to be clear and concise so I decided to write some bullet points with short cues to help my memory. They were along the lines of; Talk about the severity, Talk about non-sense mutations and mention current life expectancies. After hastily composing myself with a quick sip from a nearby *Pepsi Max* I proceeded to record.

It seemed to last for hours but those three minutes were soon over. I managed to sound coherent (talking can make my voice very breathy). One part still annoys me about two minutes in; I lost my train of thought whilst explaining the condition and for what seemed like agonising seconds I struggled to find the word "severity!" The rest of the video went really well and I remembered all I had learnt about mutations and some of the more specific disease details I wasn't aware of. An example being that I didn't know thirty percent of DMD patients suffer from some sort of non progressive developmental delay (although not mentioned as part of my video). I ended with these fighting words; "I'll live till whatever I live too, I'm not gunna just say oh I'm that age let's snuff it like..."

Not long after my production, I setup a *YouTube* account and uploaded my first video on the twelfth of July. It was not until the sixteenth (two days after my birthday) that I uploaded my DMD video; not expecting much to happen. At first I could see the views ticking over every week at about ten to twenty. I then started to get the messages and feedback and it has always been overwhelmingly positive and encouraging. I get messages from concerned people who have sons, brothers and relatives with DMD. I've had comments from other guys living with DMD; it's always good to connect with likeminded people. To date and for me the most unexpected comments I get are from medical students; I've talked to trainee physiotherapists, genetics students and nursing graduates amongst others.

I never once thought I would attract the medical world because I wasn't sure my knowledge was that good. I suppose I gave an account that both describes the condition like a textbook and crucially gives the visible human side of things. I know the breathing difficulties all to well, you can see the mini trachy sticking out of my neck, you can see the pressure mark of a ventilator mask on my nose and obviously there's the wheelchair with me sat unmoving. The devastating consequences coldly written in text are brought to life thanks to the power of the internet and *YouTube*.

Currently (as of January the first 2010) after a seeming explosion, I have over thirty thousand views! A phenomenal amount considering I never thought I'd even get a thousand. Thank you to all the watchers and if you want to see my video for yourself then here is the link:-

http://www.youtube.com/watch?v=KzftMcvplTc. I really hope it can help you and once again I want to thank all my supporters and family for being there during the rough times.

Feeling lonely one late July afternoon I decided to message a new person from the online pool league. I had met her a few days earlier whilst playing and running the odd Eight ball tournament. Her ID fascinated me by its boggling complexity, there were multiple letters set against each other. We got briefly chatting and she seemed lovely with the odd funny sarcastic remark thrown in too; like some kind of beautiful rebel. I had missed her in the pool room over the next couple of days so I fired up *Yahoo* messenger and added her complicated ID. Not long after she accepted my invite I tentatively typed a brief "hello" message out to her. She answered me back quickly and I suppose that's the day we became proper friends.

She was from the East coast of America and had long dark hair and expressive eyes. We immediately connected on a musical level; she had great taste in the kind of trance music I loved. We both listened to a lot and she introduced me to other rock bands and even one beautiful song with religious connotations. I showed her some of the British bands I knew and loved like the *Stereophonics* and *Radiohead*. *YouTube* was great for finding new songs and we'd show each other loads of different music and then see what each other thought. It was great fun experimenting with different genres and to find some surprises along the way. For instance she led me to the song *Heartbeats* preformed by

*The Knife*, which was used by another artist on a *Sony* television advert.

On a few occasions we spoke on the messenger's conference call system. It was fabulous to hear another person, she sounded very sweet with her northern states accent strongly sounding out. As ever I worried that she wouldn't be able to understand my Welsh accent but luckily there were no problems. Although I had confused her by saying I lived in a terraced house, the poor girl had visions of my house being on something like those Japanese rice terraces! I forgot that they have different ways of saying things in America, so I quickly corrected myself saying they are houses built close together. We sometimes talked about the weather over there and what music gigs she had attended.

Most of the time we just talked on the messenger sometimes for hours chatting about varied things. At that time she was studying to go into part of the medical world so I would often ask how long until her semester finished. She sometimes asked questions about my disease which I was happy to answer. I like people trying to know more about Duchenne Muscular Dystrophy because it seems hardly anyone in the general populace has heard of it. She wanted to know if I could still feel even though I was getting more and more paralysed. I indeed do still feel although it's a royal pain when something is aching or needing to be scratched! When I get extreme back ache whilst sitting in my chair, I need to call my mother and she repositions me using my hoist. What takes five seconds for the non disabled, takes me ten minutes of re-jigging! I've just got to make sure I get placed in my chair correctly.

Over August we were becoming much closer, there wasn't a day we weren't chatting. That's when I had to go and ruin it for myself! I developed a huge crush on her and decided that I had to tell her or I'd go insane not knowing how she felt. I was nervous, excited and a bit anxious as I told her about my crush and my feelings for her. She replied saying she knew I had a crush on her because she could tell by the messages and the way we talked/typed everyday. Then came the crushing news, she didn't share my feelings, saying she didn't "like me like that, it's more of a friendship thing…" I didn't know what to say as I thought we really connected and understood each other but it turned out she didn't feel the same about me. I was so gutted and felt so stupid.

I could feel myself starting to get hot and embarrassed having to fight back some warm tears. After this rejection we never really had the same level of connection. Perhaps she didn't want me to think anything was potentially blooming again. We're still good friends but I do miss what we had over that summer as I've never been so connected to a young lady before. I suppose that in the cold light of day I realize if we had dated I might have had to wait a long time to see her, much like how things ended with Miss C. Also like Miss C I didn't want my new lady friend to have to give up her potential career and sacrifice so much for me. Still I felt like my heart was broken, truly human feelings are the most strong and peculiar things to deal with. It seems doubly so for a person with DMD.

The immediate week after my rejection I dropped back down to the depths of depression. I cried so much whilst I sat typing messages to other people I was feeling so dejected and lost. Why is it I keep falling for ladies so far away? It kept breaking my heart thinking about the three recently failed attempts at relationships. Again most kinds of music set me off crying especially the ones me and my latest friend had chosen. I would wait until my mother was out of earshot before I could really let go with my eyes gently streaming and wracked with quiet sobs. Most of the time I tried to stay calm in front of my family because I didn't want them to see my tears and think I was being overly dramatic.

In the calm quiet moments of the day I would do that most dreaded of things; thinking. I thought I might never find love as all of my attempts so far had gone horribly wrong. I didn't know what to do next if I thought I was going to fall in love again. I was scared I'd fall in love with another faraway girl, so from then on in I found it hard to truly be myself in front of the lady friends I knew. If anyone started to show any hint of an interest in me I would baulk often changing subjects. I felt I had given up on girls and love, increasingly becoming used to or even resigned to not finding anyone. Don't get me wrong I certainly still want a companion but I had become wary.

Right now I am very keen to find that special lover but, I'm still fearful and have a foreboding about truly opening up to people I may want to be with. I'm so worried about yet more rejection that I find it hard trusting my feelings. It has led me to think whenever

I meet a new lady friend, is there a possibility that this someone loves me? At the back of mind I often hear, "No they can't be interested in you, don't be silly!" and "Of course they don't!" It's very hard not to keep doubting myself but I am trying because my time is fast running out. I certainly don't want to die never experiencing true love and the possibility of my own children. If sadly I don't make it then my faith promises greater things to come.

Somehow my sadness began to lift a couple of weeks later, throwing myself into my art and into pool I started to see the lighter side of life. My positivity flooded back as I laughed and joked with all my pool buddies and the small band of *Deviantart* friends I started to make. I just didn't feel like being depressed anymore I was wasting energy moping around thinking about the end. Relationships and my own mortality were just cruel distractions I didn't want to keep dragging up. Instead I just looked around for happier pursuits, including games and interesting chat rooms. I started watching the television more getting interested in my favourite subjects of science and history.

I thought at long last I was feeling like my old self of a few years prior. I was most happy entertaining myself by singing along to my favourite songs. Thrashing out as much artwork as I could manage and playing lots of online games. I retreated into my own world not worrying about my feelings just staying calm and so I thought in control of my destiny. Cruelly this was the exact time my DMD decided to get worse still. It's an awful conveyer belt of getting worse every year, every week, every month and every hour. I sometimes really wish for an emergency stop button; a big red STOP button so I can gather myself or just simply take a vacation. I was happy but now anxiety and worry were creeping back in to my life, it was yet another test of my resolve.

September 2007 felt like the worse month of my life! After a severe and debilitating bout of constipation which included a visit to my GP and some very strong laxatives, I started to feel generally unwell and sweaty. I thought sure I was having fluttery feelings in my heart (palpitations). I thought not much of it; perhaps all my pushing had caught up with me as I got so tired fighting my bowels. These palpitations felt awful as if my heart was in overdrive going well over one hundred beats per minute. I tried altering my drinks to see if it was caffeine related but that did nothing for me. I was starting to get worried as this progressed I even asked my mother to check my pulse, but she couldn't tell what was happening as she carefully felt my arm.

Then the palpitations got more frequent, not even the overnight use of my ventilator calmed me. In the mornings within minutes my hands would start pouring with sweat and I would sit in bed panting while my mother got me up. Sitting on the toilet was nigh on impossible as I would get extremely breathless and sweaty in my hoist. I would shout at my mother, "Get me off! Get me off! I can't breathe, please hurry up!" I could see black spots in front of my eyes and very nearly fainted as my heart would try to hammer its way out. Getting back in my chair was such a relief but my poor mother would be exhausted after all my shouts, gasps and hurrying. I knew something was majorly wrong because I was not my normal calm self; I thought I was dying!

It was now consuming my time as I was constantly looking forward to sleep and my ventilator. I would rush my mother to switch it on so I could at least get some rest after long sweaty and panic filled days. My father could tell I was in distress when I started needing the ventilator in the daytime which was unheard of for me. I couldn't even enjoy the television as my heart would be a constant distraction. I tried everything to keep myself occupied I found painting the only calming thing as well as closing my eyes to sleep. It felt like only a matter of time until my heart finally gave up the ghost. My mother being extremely worried got me to contact my respiratory team in Llandough explaining my symptoms.

Their reply was for me to go to straight to Llandough so they could evaluate my condition. My father had to take me on his own the next day which was a Wednesday. My mother had to stay home while some work was being done to my lift. The drive down was agonising as my breathlessness was coming on thick and fast. I was sweating profusely but it was an awful cold sweat that made me look ghostly white. As we headed nearer to Llandough I could see the black spots in front of my eyes and I had gotten so quiet just willing myself to be well. After my father parked the van we rushed into the lung function department where I was quickly shepherded in to a side room. My father asked me if I needed the *Nippy* on and I gratefully accepted as my heart and lungs burned and ached for air.

As the cooling air hit me I immediately gasped in relief as everyone looked on with worried faces. A few minutes later a cardiologist comes in to check on me, a nice chap called Dr. Yousuf. He tried talking to me (but it's next to impossible to be heard on a face mask) to see how I was doing. Instead my father told him my worrying symptoms. After a conference with his registrar he approached my father and I and said; "Your last scan from 2001 indicates a problem developing in you're heart…" He then went on to mention a few drugs he would like to try me on and said I needed to stay in hospital. I was astonished that if my scan showed trouble in 2001 why wait until 2007 to treat me. Again the failure of the NHS to monitor my condition meant I was receiving reactionary medicine once more!

I was booked in to a special side room on the old Victorian west ward 4 in Llandough. I was painfully moved on to a bed by a hoist that didn't suit my needs which bruised me in some *very* delicate places! Then in came my respiratory doctor and examined me, he was worried by a fold line on my back which he thought was a scar but that turned out to be nothing. Next he was concerned with my weight as I looked really scrawny and bony; I was weighed in a weighing chair and found to be only six stone four pounds (eighty eight pounds). My immediate concern was my heart and I was still having trouble with constipation. Dr Gelder (respiratory doctor) then told me I was going to be put on more laxatives and ominously, examined!

Two minutes later a fairly senior nurse came in with a rubber glove and a tray of *Microlax* enemas. I was nervous of what was coming next, thinking I'd jump to the proverbial ceiling! She skilfully placed her finger where it was so not wanted but she had to check what was going on. While she was examining me she kept talking about how the rectum works! I thought this is hardly the time or the place to be talking about reservoirs in my back passage. Thankfully it was soon over and after using two micro enemas I was allowed to lie back in peace. Apparently everything was "soft" so they were proceeding with a top down approach of oral laxatives. I was keen to forget that ever happened but we still joke about reservoirs even now.

The new drugs for my heart were called *Digoxin* (derived from foxglove to control palpitations), *Carvedilol* (a beta blocker to control heart rate), *Lisinopril* an ACE inhibitor (very much like a beta blocker) and *Furosemide* (a diuretic). Later in the coming years I would be given *Spironolactone* (another type of milder diuretic). I needed all the drugs in liquid form because of my even worsening swallow (that has steadily declined since I was nineteen). The only exception being *Carvedilol* which has never been given to me in liquid form, so I have to suck it until it dissolves. All of the medicines taste horrible but I have gotten used to them. It took a good three to four days until I felt the full benefits of the drugs slowing and easing my heart as the hours passed by.

It was immensely relieving to finally not be sweaty or struggling to breathe. After just five days I was nearly ready to be sent home with my ensemble of new drugs. By a stroke of chance I discovered some food I could eat on the second day I was admitted. I was discussing with a nurse about my eating difficulties and they suggested that I try the puree menu the hospital had. One funny memory I have was upon seeing a pureed corn beef hash. I enquired "this is a normal piece of meat, how am I supposed to eat it?" After my first mouthful I had realised how foolish I was as the meat thinned out and turned out to be liquidised. I was immensely happy as the delicious tastes passed my mouth and for the first time in years I felt hungry!

By day seven I was discharged and feeling a lot better. The pureed food I found by chance had given me more energy and the heart drugs settled my anxieties greatly. My bowels released their horrible grip on me as the laxatives had the desired effect on me (it's an awful part of DMD I know). I felt much more settled and calm and my ventilator use had dropped down to just mainly at night, with maybe an extra boost hour during the day. I was left to return home with a bag of new medicines, including four main heart drugs and two types of laxative, one daily and one for emergencies. My stomach must be like a vat in the *ICI* plant with all the lotions and potions I now take. It's worth it though to feel well again at least for the time being.

It was an excellent feeling coming back home to the normality of broadband and my beloved *Pepsi Max*. The first change for my mother was the way she made my meals. My father had bought a *Phillips* hand blender that my mother could use to blitz all my food. After many nights of trial and error she could liquidise a few different vegetables and the contents of a *Fray Bentos* flat pie. It was a strange feeling to swallow liquidised carrots and cauliflower; I got all these tastes but not the textures you would expect. It was fantastic to finally have vegetables after many years choking down oven fritters and fish not feeling hungry at all. Another change for me was the need to have a wheelchair headrest to ease the pressure on my neck. My father adapted the bog standard NHS headrest I had, using a square piece of high density foam and a "G" clamp to hold it. I love it and still need it now.

I was restless through December as pool had became harder to play (my hands and fingers got too achy) and I started to think of my heart more in between typing and shooting. Even though I felt better with the new heart drugs, some days I was feeling better than others. I felt more fragile and worn out as even light tasks would put a strain on me. DMD always tightens its grip every year and every month, it is utterly oppressive and gives me constant worries and a few desperate thoughts. To combat the relentless nature of this disease I try to throw myself into many varied things from music listening, game playing, art, pool and anything else that interested me. I decided that I wanted to give something back in my latest endeavour for all the likeminded lads my age living with DMD.

I gave something back by making my own website called *DuchenneMen* which can be found here at http://duchennemen.net16.net or on most search engines. It was a hard slog trying to teach myself the internet language called hyper text transfer protocol. Most commands need to be written in between special bracketed control letters. For example to add a web address you need to set it up like so; <a href=http://example.com> example.com</a>

There are various commands that you would need to learn to set your own site up, but I found a dearth of information on many different websites and from a few friends I knew on the internet. After a few weeks hard work I had setup a basic blue background and a few buttons or links to other pages; I was planning to produce new web pages using my original code as a guide. I had painted the background and made up the button icons myself along with any other images I needed. I even came up with the blue and red logo of *DuchenneMen* that proudly sits atop the homepage.

I setup the site aimed at giving men with DMD a voice because a lot of sites are too parent oriented and focus at the newly diagnosed younger boys. That's necessary and quite understandable because DMD takes a heavy toll on the parents, but I really wanted to give us so called 'older' sufferers a voice. I found hardly any sites aimed specifically at us so I took matters into my own hands. I have topics ranging from heart troubles, mini- tracheotomies, nutrition and adult issues. Recently I made a section called 'Interviews' in which I asked a group of men living with Duchenne to answer a few probing questions. I got a good response getting three other guys to tell me what they did all day and their general feelings about love and the future of DMD.

I have a section dedicated to my own thoughts and feelings that I update every two months. I call this my

'Editorial'. It's like my personal journal as well as an extra place for information that doesn't fit in the other sections of the site. Views of my site have been intermittent but I try to generate more by linking to the homepage of many different sites that I'm a part of including; social network sites, *DeviantArt*, Pool and many others. Finding a free website host was quite easy, I had to simply enter 'free website hosting' in a search engine and up popped hundreds of links. I was careful to check out the small print to see what I was or wasn't allowed to do and crucially how much space you could use on the internet (bandwidth). I'm really happy with the place I found though.

The first few months of 2008 went quickly and pretty much normally (normal for me at least considering my condition). My website had consumed a vast amount of time and was now beginning to look a lot more useful. I added my successful DMD video from the year before and a description of what Duchenne is. I was enjoying my new pureed diet so much so that I was eating too many carrots! I had developed an orange/red complexion and looked really awful. After a blood test preformed at a regular appointment my respiratory consultant informed me that I had something he hadn't seen in many years that being carrot anaemia! Immediately I was advised to vastly cut down the amount of carrots I was consuming. My mother did this straight away and I now only have them once a week.

During May however because of my continued eating difficulties my respiratory consultant thought I should have a feeding tube put into my stomach. Quickly without my knowledge he arranged a hospital stay to put it in. I was surprised by the speed I was rushed in to the hospital and as a result it was one of the worst hospital stay's I have ever had. I require a lot of equipment, my mobile hoist which only fits my sling (unlike the hospitals own inappropriate hoist), my suction machine, my suction catheters, my suction gloves, my mattress (the hospital couldn't provide me with an appropriate air mattress, they had none free for me, even though they knew I was coming), my wheelchair and my ventilator.

All this requires a side room which I got the last few times I was in hospital. Not this time however, I was placed on a general men's ward which had very little space for my equipment. A lot of it was stowed in various rooms all over the ward. I require twenty four hour care and vigilance due to my DMD induced paralysis and the condition itself. This means my mother has to stay with me incase I need suction (which has to be done immediately), feeding, bathing/washing (even though the bath room was inaccessible; she had to use a flannel) and anything else I needed. The nurses just did not seem to understand this; they told my mother to sleep in a room one hundred yards away and to leave me the call button. My mother had to explain that due to my severe weakness and hand deformities (contractures) I was unable to even hold the call button, let alone press it.

When it was time to sleep, I had to be hoisted into bed in front of eight or so other men, losing my dignity in the process as I was undressed ready for sleeping. We tried closing the curtain but it impeded the hoist's movement so it had to be opened. Once in bed at around ten I was stopped from eating until the procedure, which was promised to be the following morning. It was extremely cold that night and I was shivering under the sheets, I even had to put my own fleece blankets on. My mother had to sleep upright in a chair using her coat as a blanket, unsurprisingly she got no sleep. In a side room we would have had room for a small bed my mother could have used to sleep in.

The next day I had to be put back in my chair, (again losing my dignity). Then I waited to be called down to the day theatre. Nine o'clock passed and then three o'clock by which time I was struggling to breathe having no energy caused by the lack of food. I had to go on my ventilator most of the day until finally at 4:30 pm I was called down to theater! I was desperately hungry and felt like I had zero energy, this led to me becoming terrified as my breathing seemed to be giving out on me. I was also scared by the fact I wasn't allowed painkillers or a local anesthetic, due to the risks associated with DMD I suppose.

In theatre I had a numbing spray applied at the back of my throat which affected my chest secretions but I could not talk to warn people. Next the surgeons tried to lay me on my back but in a cruel twist my earlier unoperated scoliosis prevented me from laying flat. I didn't know I couldn't lie as flat as they needed me. The whole procedure was called off after this and I was rushed back up to the ward to use my ventilator, I thought I would pass out by then. An hour later I came off the ventilator to speedily eat some pureed food and I immediately started to feel better, able to breathe on my own until bed time that night. In the confusion after the failed procedure I was told I could go home, then told to stay and then told to go home again. After being messed about so much I decided to go home.

The next day at home Llandough's dietician rang to say I should have stayed in the hospital as she was worried about my weight. Eventually she referred me to a lovely new local dietician, who immediately put me on food supplements (both milk based) and boosted the types of pureed food I could have (namely by adding cheese, milk and thickeners to my food). Luckily this worked and I regained three stone over the coming year, annoyingly no previous dieticians or doctors had suggested adequate supplements before my nightmare stay in the hospital. I had no dietician monitoring me prior to this hospital stay apart from one who wasn't really of any use and seemed to forget about me.

June was a month that changed a lot in my life; it gave me purpose and a solid determination I didn't think I had. Checking my emails one day I came across an email from a lady named Julia. She was wondering if I had heard of a charity called *Action Duchenne* that was aiming to bring about publicity and an eventual treatment for DMD. I had heard of the charity and was not really sure if I could fit in because it seemed parent oriented but I hadn't looked in to it thoroughly. The most surprising thing was that she wanted to visit me at home, I thought in relation to my website which is where she found my email address. I was eager to meet her because no one had ever wanted to visit me at home in many years. I wasn't afraid of meeting her because

*Action Duchenne* seemed to be an honest and very trustworthy place.

She came on a beautiful bright summer day wearing a long flowing skirt, her hair fluttering in the breeze. At first there was an awkward silence as I had no idea what this meeting was really about. The meeting wasn't much to do with my site; that was just our introduction point. Julia brought two large booklets that had a wealth of cool information about *Action Duchenne* and the disease itself. After my initial quietness we got chatting, she was determined and funny. She wanted a treatment for Duchenne to be found and was fully committed to that cause. I was quickly getting interested in the idea of helping out. She was keen to get me on board and recommended I join a registry that DMD patients could go on to find out their eligibility for clinical trials (http://www.dmdregistry.org/).

All too soon Julia had to leave ready to catch her train back to England. My mother and I both thought she was lovely and had a genuine caring nature. We struck up a friendship on the *Action Duchenne* website and a popular social network site. I signed up to *Action Duchenne*, thinking how lucky and apt it was that she had found me through my website. My misgivings about it being overly parent oriented were unfounded as one of the main protagonists was a young man living with DMD. He was only a couple of years younger than me and is called Carl. I was so glad this wasn't just a parent only site but we sufferers were welcome too. After making my introduction, I was greeted very kindly finding a wide mix of people from all backgrounds. The sense of community I felt was palpable. I was finally part of a family that understood my needs.

Over the course of the month Julia would ring me a lot seeing if I was ok and wondering how I could help. I told her of my artwork skills, she was intrigued by this fact. We formulated a plan to make some postcards that *Action Duchenne* could sell to raise much needed funds. I picked some of my best designs to date, including a red vase, a drawing of a *VW* van, a pocket watch design, a flaming leaf, a beach at sunrise and a drawing of a midnight blue pendant. I sent them all along to Julia and she loved them, it wasn't long until they were up and running and selling well. They are sold at the annual international *Action Duchenne* conference where parents and sufferers meet with scientists in London. Unfortunately I am unable to go because it's a distance I can't make as I need a load of equipment and my pureed food.

As my twenty fourth birthday approached I had developed a fire in my belly to finally see the end of DMD. *Action Duchenne* had a wealth of information and I found out so much. I could see the parents going through it, struggling with new diagnosis and generally being understandably upset. I would see photos of strapping young kids that I knew would face the same difficulties as me. It breaks my heart that more boys and men are going to die unless we keep up the pressure on the NHS and the government.

Shamefully the government health department had woefully underfunded research in DMD, only spending about two million pounds over a twenty year period! *Action Duchenne* lobby the governments of England, Wales, Scotland and Northern Ireland on these issues every year, and also pump in vastly more funds than had ever gone to DMD before. Finally scientists can try to find treatments in humans, instead of theorising and using a test mouse called the "MDx Mouse model". We are people not mice after all and happily many trials are starting to use humans but as of yet the cure is still elusive. The battle will continue and I hope to be a part in finally ridding this world of DMD once and for all.

# Age twenty four to age twenty five

In this the final chapter of my book I am going to explain my current thoughts, feelings and activities under the following sub headings. I will discuss my current medical and home condition, my feelings on sexuality, my artwork and writing, music, more on my work with *Action Duchenne*, the family and lastly the future.

## Current condition

In the last year and a half my condition has declined; whilst that is to be expected with DMD, it never gets any easier. My hands have continued to weaken and that has effectively stopped me from playing online pool anymore. Moving my finger from the left mouse button to the right takes so much effort that I'm too tired to enjoy playing. The other way to play involving the on screen keyboard requires multiple fast clicks which again wear me out. If I do pop in to pool it's only generally to chat to some of my old friends but they aren't often in there. Chatting is fine but the whole point of an online pool room is to eventually play the game. Naturally this has meant I've lost interest, so I try to catch up with friends on *Yahoo* messenger or on social network sites instead.

The rest of my body hasn't been moveable for many years. My neck has gotten so weak that it can barely support my head. My head leans to the right and it seems many other Muscular Dystrophy patients' heads do this too. My father has made me a foam support for my standard head rest so I can relieve the pressure on my neck. I get other aches and pains daily, my wrist can hurt using my light mouse, my back hurts everyday either in my bed or in my chair and I can get elbow pain. Often I get chest pains when my heart is misbehaving either because I'm late taking my medicines or it's the cardiomyopathy itself. My lungs only hurt when they are full of mucus; drowning in your own secretions is certainly painful; luckily suctioning relieves that pain quickly. I don't tend to complain about the pain because I've gotten used to something always aching. If it's excruciating then I have to ask my mother to move me into a better position or I'll ask for a painkiller (very rarely).

Another alarming change has been the deterioration of my breathing. I have quickly gone from roughly ten hours at night and three hours in the day to eighteen hours per day on my ventilator. This has impacted heavily on my daily living as I have to make sure I'm near my ventilator. I recently needed to upgrade to a more portable unit. It's called an *Elisee* which can be found on many intensive care units. It took me six months of hard work to get it off Llandough hospital. I had a few run-ins' with some of the staff who told me unless there was a medical need to change from my current ventilators it wouldn't happen. I had two large *Nippy* ventilators; one was a backup for my main night ventilator. Fearing that these bulky machines would mean staying at home indefinitely, I emailed Paula the senior nurse with my concerns and eventually got the newer machine (with a bit of help from *Action Duchenne* too).

The scary thing about my declining breathing was the speed at which it recently changed. Whilst eating a meal one Saturday evening I began to feel extremely breathless and very anxious. My swallowing which is bad normally turned much worse to the point where I thought I'd choke. I was very worried because I had similar symptoms when my heart was first diagnosed with cardiomyopathy. For a few nights I thought I was actually going to have a heart attack! My mother even had to spend a nights' vigil reassuring me that everything would be alright and to keep my faith in the Lord.

The following Wednesday I had a clinic visit scheduled, so I went to Llandough to see what was wrong with me. I had various tests on my heart all whilst wearing my ventilator and I had a separate twenty four hour heart trace. After a few days wait I got the results back. It showed that my current drugs were controlling my heart just fine and that it wasn't a cardiac problem affecting my breathing. I was shocked because I was convinced it was my heart causing all my recent breathing difficulties. My respiratory team still don't know what is causing my recent decline but the only option left to me is to suppose that it's my DMD getting worse. That probably being the case means there's nothing I can do to change it. I have to face the rest of my life needing to use a ventilator over eighteen hours a day and likely right up to twenty four hours.

Another major concern for me has been the amount of chest suction I now require. For about a year now I've been using around twenty catheters a day. It wouldn't be so bad if it took a few seconds to get through all those plastic life sparing tubes. Unfortunately each session of suction involving about five catheters can take up to two hours. It's extremely tiring for both me and my mother (or caregiver). For me its tough trying to muster enough of a cough to get the secretions sucked up (because of my very weak almost non existent cough). For my mother or caregiver it must be tiring constantly moving a catheter up and down my trachea. I found the most effective way of moving secretions is to hold my breath briefly then exhale while the suction machine does its thing; it feels like a poor mans cough but it works for me.

The most draining and depressing part of chest suction for me is the fact that there's always more mucus likely to develop. After the usual hour or two of suction in the morning/afternoon I'm exhausted and hungry. After breakfast and my medication I'm put on my ventilator and think about using my computer. An hour or so later I feel the telltale signs that my chest is filling up again; one slight turn of my head or if some saliva tickles my throat, I'm coughing or choking again! It's so relentless the way the mucus keeps attacking my lungs; everyday I'm faced with long hours of coughing, spluttering and holding my breath just to get through.

The moments before bed are the worst because both my mother and I are tired and fed up of the daily slog. I'm often asking myself 'why?' during those times, but I grit my teeth and get it over with; then it's into bed for a restless sleep. I'm always concerned the mucus will come back while I sleep on my ventilator so I try to keep my bed as upright as possible to avoid this. The downsides however are that my back can hurt (I can get excruciating nerve pain) and that it's not an entirely sleep conducive position. Usually I drift off at about four or five in the morning escaping all my chest and disease worries before it all begins again at twelve. Some days I feel like being left there, that I cannot be bothered to deal with another day busting my gut to move secretions that will only come back! My mother opens my door however and I just try to shake off that thought and wake up.

The suction machine I use now is called a *SAM 12*; it's a huge bulky box that has a strong suction action. Strength of suction is measured in millimetres of mercury (mmHg). It can reach up to six hundred and fifty mmHg which feels nice and strong while it works away. It's not the first suction machine I've had, for many years I had a machine called an *LSU* which was a small bright blue and yellow machine that could reach five hundred and fifty mmHg. It worked fine up until 2008, but as my suctioning needs were increasing it couldn't keep up. On three separate occasions it broke down leaving me without any suction machine! The third brake down happened at nine in the evening which meant my mother had to make an emergency call to our district nurses. They managed to find me the *SAM 12* I now use.

I was glad they found me the *SAM 12* because it felt so much stronger and able to deal with my needs than the *LSU*. I thought this would now be the machine they (the health authority) would continue letting me use.

When the *SAM 12* was due to be serviced I hit major problems getting a replacement. The health authority wanted me to go back to using the *LSU* which is totally inappropriate for my increased needs. I refused to let them take the *SAM 12* off me and decided to ring the head of purchasing at the local hospital. I was then told that the *SAM 12* was to be made obsolete! Naturally I was scared to death that I'd be left with a machine that couldn't handle my needs, which would put my life in jeopardy and this in turn made me feel very low.

Determined not to give up I got an address from my uncle that led to a person at the very top of the hospital complaints department. I wrote a passionate letter detailing all that had gone on, from the broken *LSU's* right up to the apparent withdrawing of the *SAM 12*. I wrote how worried and terrified I was, that I'd be left in a worse situation with an inadequate machine. A few days later I received an answer saying they would investigate my concerns within twenty days. True to their word I received a phone call from the lady I wrote too. Her answer was that there had been a mix up, in actuality the *SAM 12* units were not being scrapped but just that the supplier was changing. The lady apologized for the stress caused to me and promised that this would not happen again. Hopefully that will be the end of that but it was a very stressful six months fighting to get it sorted.

All my daily troubles and the often immovable and stubborn NHS can make my emotional state very changeable. Depression has been a big part of my life and many major periods have been written about in this book. Often it's after relationship problems; which seem to have a keen knack of making me focus on things I cannot do. It's an awful feeling trapped in a failing body, watching it slowly waste and die in front of you. There's nothing that can be changed by being constantly upset and tearful even though it feels like I'm a mere layer of varnish away from that. I simply haven't got the tears to cry for the twenty odd years I've been alive.

Somehow I've developed a strength or resolve just to carry on with a positive demeanour. It is so hard to keep the 'brave' face on; it's as if God has just given me enough to get through each problem.

There's an added pressure I seem to get from other people; because they mostly see the positive side of me, I get the feeling I'm expected to always be positive. Some days I want to scream and shout at how tough things are but I'm worried that I will somehow let people down who look up to me. Lots of my friends are mothers of other boys with Duchenne, and I know they appreciate my seemingly positive attitude the most. Other men my age with Duchenne also sometimes make me feel, that I'm letting the side down when I'm feeling negative. It always feels like we DMD sufferers and families have to always mask our true feelings because other people don't understand us. It's time we showed the world what it is really like to live with DMD, otherwise how else will the people understand. If the world truly knew then we perhaps could get the real support and change we need.

What gets me through each day is my faith, the family and friends I have who understand everything DMD, my art, my writing and listening to music. If I don't keep my mind focussed on these other things, I'll always wander back into the darker, fearful and worrying parts of my consciousness. Being dependant on others for absolutely *everything* makes you worry who will keep looking after you're needs, who will keep my chest clear and will my ventilator continue working. These are worries non disabled people think nothing of, a mere decision to them could be potentially life threatening for me.

Let's take climate change for example, *Greenpeace* seem to want every one to stop using electricity. It's easy for them to pitch a tent and live up a tree getting closer to nature, but for the dependant people like me we need our wheelchairs and ventilators charged and reliable power for suction machines, hoists, beds, mattresses and food blenders. The drastic changes proposed by environmentalists and governments never factor in these problems. They just talk about 'keeping the lights on' but for me and others in similar situations it is a question of life or death. I'm not surprised given all this that a proportion of DMD sufferers develop mental health issues. This probably is another reason we (DMD families) need to tell the world of our problems.

## My Sexuality;

A difficult topic for me to discuss is my sexuality. I'm a straight twenty five year old guy writing this. I really appreciate the female form and I like all its curves and indents; it reminds me of a tapestry in silk. A lot of women and other men seem to think people in wheelchairs don't think about sex or worse still are "Asexual" i.e. oblivious and unaffected by the needs and urges of sexuality. This attitude is often reinforced by so called healthcare professionals. I just want to say this is not the case; I am a 'normal' man in that department.

I get pent up sexual frustrations like any other man. It's not a case that I can go boxing or take a cold shower. I can't even get a girlfriend, let alone make intimate decisions over reasoned discussions. With television and other media throwing love, companionship and all the kissing around me I can't escape my frustrations. As a man paralysed by DMD I cannot please a woman in a way that could possibly satisfy either of us.

Women don't seem to be interested in me like that anyway. I can understand why, my body looks so different from the norm. I have deformed hands that look like fists unable to be straightened; I wonder how I am supposed to 'feel' all the curves I like. My leg joints can't take pressure on them. I would need to be carefully put in my bed and have some sort of contortionist woman to find a comfortable position. I can't think of many women wanting to do that (I certainly don't want to pay anyone either). A few people have told me that this person exists, it just doesn't help me. Peoples' throw away statements just make me feel worse and more inadequate. I will supposedly "find someone who doesn't care about what I can't do" and that "if I keep looking I'll find her" or even "I believe there's someone out there for everyone".

Well there isn't much left I can do, I'm sure a winning personality won't please a lady all of the time and I want to offer more! I have immense trouble looking for potential partners; going out for me involves a military procedure of arranging transport, dressing, ventilators and the suction machine for my chest. That's exhausting and by the end of it I'd only be out an hour hardly enough time to be finding a lover. I suppose the old "someone for everyone" thing might work if you live seventy years but that's not looking realistic for me at the moment.

To combat my frustrations I'll admit to watching 'adult' videos and the like and everything that a man does while watching. I find that extremely difficult to do lately, I can't move my hands, legs or anything. I've found a novel way to 'help myself' so to speak. Sadly the way DMD works there'll be a time when I'm too weak to do anything like that even if wanted too. Following a recent religious revival however I no longer choose to 'help myself' but want to wait until I find someone special even though that is difficult, there is more to life than sex I suppose and I believe greater things await us. It doesn't mean I don't ever want these experiences mind you.

To those who think I'm morally wrong for previously using 'adult' entertainment, I say try living your whole life without touch or sex. Try living where everyone thinks you cannot even have sexual feelings.

Then ask yourself if you wouldn't fall into watching 'adult' entertainment. I hope my family don't think any less of me for the things I've written here. I'm sure they will be fine, but I find this topic so difficult to talk to them about. I feel quite isolated as there's no-one else to talk too. If I find a girlfriend, I'll want companionship, cosy nights in front of the television, plenty of hugging and after discussion we might have sex or I'll wait until an unlikely wedding. It would have to be a different kind of love making but if that cannot be achieved; I'd at least want to be open about sexuality.

I would be happy to be hugged and touched. As humans we crave touch. It feels like torture not being touched. If a man isn't supposed to be an island, why do I feel like one? Very few people can understand what all this truly feels like, apart from my fellow DMD peers. I do hope I've given you an insight. Just to reiterate that those of us in wheelchairs are not asexual and do think of and enjoy sex. I know of a few DMD guys married and having their own families in a few different countries. I'm always hopeful that I'll find Miss Right but it is certainly a very difficult task!

## Art and writing;

I'd now like to show you a small fraction of my art and writing from the three and a half years I've been on *DeviantArt*. I'll provide an explanation below each piece and the year they were made. I've explored many varied styles and don't really like to pin myself to any particular genre of art as you will see.

The above piece is entitled **Sunrise beach,** I made this back in 2006. After the earlier digital palette knife beach painting I received some uplifting and helpful comments. I took the positive criticism on board and produced this picture. I took roughly an hour to complete it using digital oils and various coarse blending tools provided in *Painter IX*. I've always liked sunsets and sunrises and had a really pleasurable time making

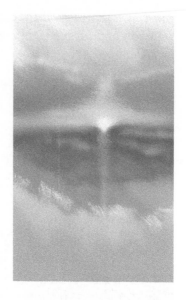

this. It just goes to show how positive reinforcement can lead to even greater things. Lastly you've got to admit that God's Earth is a wonderful place to live.

This piece is entitled **Self Portrait Ian;** I painted this again back in 2006. It's painted from the photo that made Miss B 'feel sick'. It shows me leaning against my pillow in bed whilst on my full face mask. It's one of my first portraits and it took a lot of experimenting getting my face pigmentation right. For me the eyes stand out the

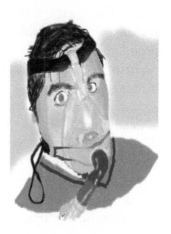

most, it's almost as if they are piercing but at the same time soft and caring. I still use the same face mask at night as is depicted above.

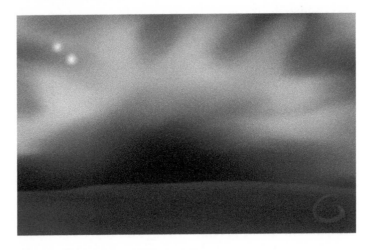

This is my most viewed painting on *DeviantArt* (I currently have over twenty thousand views), it is entitled **Aurora Borealis Wallpaper**. I produced this in 2007. The northern lights have always fascinated me; it's amazing that billions of interacting particles can produce something so beautiful. I just had to try and capture it, I mixed blues and greens with a coarse blender then blurred the resultant image to make it appear ethereal. I added the green hill to give it some scale and depth. Finally I sprayed digital white paint to illustrate the stars in outer space. I added the brightest stars to complete the picture. Recently I signed it with my new big G signature, which has always been my ID on *Deviantart*. It has 'wallpaper' in its title because it was specifically intended to be used as a desktop computer background.

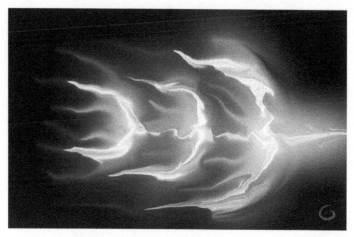

This piece is called **Fireleaf** produced in 2008. I find the patterns and dancing of flames fascinating and I believe it's one of the toughest things to capture artistically. This was my attempt at emulating nature; I used a tool that distorted the colours and bright glows you painted down into many varied shapes. I 'pulled' the oranges and reds into the interesting pattern you can see. It turned out better than I could have imagined and indeed looks like a leaf made of fire.

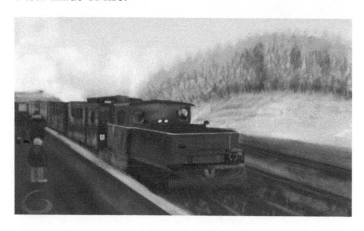

This piece is called **Winter Train** and was made at the end of 2009. I used an old photo stored on my computer that my father took, as a reference to create this piece. It's a station in Brecon which is about twenty to thirty miles away. This is a recent change in styles for me as I really wanted to get back to actually painting in a 'traditional' sense. A television programme called 'Crawshaw paints' reignited my passion for painting as the presenter showed how easy it was after all. Within *Painter IX* you have the ability to choose the 'paper' you want to use. I chose an artists rough paper and painted using digital oils. I loved painting this, my sister helped point out a few flaws and after my corrections it added an extra realism to the piece.

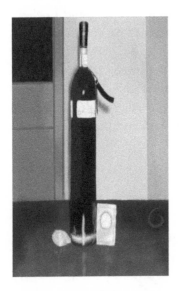

The final piece I want to share with you is called **Port and Ornaments**. This was made towards the end of 2009; I setup a still life as I hadn't ever really painted one save for a few imagined pieces. I told my mother how to arrange the above items until I was satisfied, then a reference photo was taken so I could refer to it at my leisure. It was a few hours work spread over two days. I thoroughly enjoyed mixing virtual colours and matching tones, that gorgeous port colour looked so rich. The two other items are a silver plated sea shell and a plated watch in the shape of a photo frame. I'm not entirely happy with the metal colouring but overall the piece turned out better than I thought. In fact many people have commented on *DeviantArt* that the painting looks photo realistic even though I wasn't aiming for that. God has blessed me with this artistic talent and I'm so glad to help *Action Duchenne* through my paintings.

Now I'd like to show you some of my poetry that I write whenever something catches my mind. A few poems are dedicated to DMD and have even been read out at *Action Duchenne* lobbies during 2009. Again I will explain when they were produced and my thoughts and feelings behind every piece. I got interested in poetry about two years ago after I began seeing examples on *DeviantArt* and remembering that I enjoyed poems when my old English teacher Mr. Key had set us a poetry challenge. I don't particularly follow any strict poetry rules, sometimes things rhyme sometimes they don't but it is all from the heart.

A tribute…This is a tribute to all my fallen comrades. They were not slain by weapons. Nor war wounds but still heroes to the end. Taken by the dark claw of this deadly muscle disease. They were strong to the fore. Strength to their core while all around muscles receded. They were workers, businessmen, artists and friends. An inner power of towering energy known no bounds. Great public orators letting all know their struggle to be equal. To be equal in standards of care, equal in love. Equal in society in a world not geared for them. From innocent childhood to paralysing adulthood. Misery not their style, happiness and warmth their comforter. No pity for them please. Just remember them. The brave forgotten few. Our brothers, our sons, our fathers, our friends. Taken before their time.

The poem above was written in early 2009 to highlight the plight of men and boys living with DMD. It's from a personal and broader viewpoint. It makes people think about things not normally associated with my disease, how we are sometimes fathers and lovers and family and friends and workers. I highlighted how this non disabled world isn't geared for us, in terms of complete wheelchair access and being able to eat and breathe and many other issues. It is also a tribute to all the DMD boys and men that have died but left wonderful legacies in their families lives. Finally it's a way of bringing our lives to the attention of the general population many who have never heard of Duchenne Muscular Dystrophy.

The Duchenne Soldier. O glorious band of brothers we. Fighting an enemy unseen, Unheard of. Unknown by the masses, always deadly none-the-less. We who have no choice, no Kings shilling for us. No special uniform, only a wrecked body. No regiments, no battalions, no guns, just each other. From Mother to Brother, Father to Sister. Genetic disease our conflict, our war. Will we win? - We're still waiting for the magic bullet. Paralysis the enemy tank, Lack of knowledge - a cruel propaganda. Please help! Our battle cry until our dying breath. A one hundred percent death rate, no parades for us. Just a quiet family heartbreak. This is what it means to be a Duchenne Soldier.

This poem highlights each and every person with DMD who are fighting personal battles against this disease.

I also wanted to highlight that many DMD patients die at similar ages to the soldiers who fight wars with bullets. We have no weapon or treatment to fight our war yet we just struggle on with positivity. I see an inner strength in many of my friends who are living their lives with Duchenne. I was making a statement that no-one apart from close family even know that two boys/men die from DMD every week. We fight a brave fight through many deadly situations but don't get parades or even general media coverage. When ever I do see a rare story about DMD I take an interest. The main stories here in Wales are about the non existent care offered by the health service. The poem was produced in 2009.

The unflinching hand. As I look across the room at you. I want to hold you I want to feel you. I want to feel your soft shoulders in my palms. Run my hands over your back feel every indent and fold on your gentle shoulder blades. Feel the warmth of your cheek, run my fingers over your smooth forehead. Cup your breasts in my hands feel the soft bountiful skin between my fingers. I can not do any of that for I have an unflinching hand an unmoveable body. You offer to place my hand on your pleasant surfaces.

You lift my arm in the air; my clenched hand falls limply down. I can not straighten my hand out, to do so the pain excruciating. So you run the back of my hand upon your skin, it feels numb to me I can't feel the gentle warmth it's dead to me! My unflinching hand, unmoveable body stopping me. I want to hug you; I would move my body closer look into your eyes. Give you the tell, move myself, go face to face, swoop my arms around you.

Hold you in a deep embrace melting the troubles of our world away. I'd want to kiss you, to feel your soft smooth lips caress mine, that knowing touch of love. I would smell your hair, place my head by your cheek enjoy the heady scent of lavender upon a rose. I can not do any of that for I have an unflinching hand an unmoveable body.

My body a prison, growing each day, the locks bigger by the hour. The walls close in, squeezing the life out of me; I can't see my jailor for he is invisible to me. My kryptonite, my genetic disease it grows stronger, I grow weaker. Another year alone without your touch, without your love, without ...you! All hope seems lost. The only thing keeping me going is finding that key to free me from this prison inside. Will I win or will I give in, those who know me know the answer. Those who do not, help find the key. For that is the story of me.

This is a very emotional poem for me as it highlights the difficulty of being close and intimate with a lady. Being severely weakened and having contracted fingers makes running my hand over anything impossible. I can see everywhere around me the importance of touch but I'm not able to interact with any of it. I feel great sadness about that but for my sanity I try to avoid dwelling on what I can't do. The odd pang of sadness and longing creeps in say whenever I want a hug or I see people embracing each other or if something needs to be touched (like a button or touch screen). All of this is increasingly adding to my isolation from everyday things many take for granted. Again this poem was made in 2009.

Wales the land of song. Wales the land of Welsh. Wales the land of cawl and Bara brith. Wales the land of lava bread but no volcano. Wales the land of my fathers. Wales the land of rugby tradition.

Wales the land of green valleys and snow capped mountains. Wales the land of the red dragon "Y Ddraig Goch". Wales the land of wide beaches and narrow straits. Wales the land of sheep covered hilltops. Wales the land of rain and mud.

I wrote this small poem at the turn of 2009. I love Wales as a country and enjoy the diverse culture and history we are surrounded by. It's a quick tour of my country from the mountains to the coast, from the house to the rugby pitch and from the English language to the Welsh. I'd like to speak more Welsh but I find learning languages very difficult; I'm struggling to speak anyway as my throat muscles continue to weaken. A friend on *DeviantArt* wrote her own poem on Wales and when I saw it, I was fired up with passion and just had to write my own piece.

## Music;

Music has always been in my life, around the periphery or right in the forefront. I remember singing along to the top 40 way back when "Ice, Ice baby" was popular. I used to love listening to cassette tapes on my *Sony Walkman* fast forwarding to my favourite song; sometimes I'd find the beginning of the song! I would turn the volume up and drift away into another place while my favourite artists blasted out their lyrics. I liked all sort of artists, my fathers *Star wars* soundtrack LP, Michael Jackson, A-Ha, Duran-Duran and loads of different instrumental tracks. My tastes have always been very varied and could certainly be called eclectic. Most of my early memories of music revolve around listening to the radio.

I can recall many hours listening to music while my father drove me wherever we needed to go (often hospital appointments down in Cardiff). I would sing along to music played on local commercial radios; getting mad at all the adverts taking me away from the music. At other times my father would put his cassettes on and sing loudly which would make Sian and I laugh. Sometimes I would like a particular tape my father would have on, an example being the original *Pure Moods* cassette. I loved some of the songs because they were instrumental and made me relax on long difficult journeys.

It seems when you're young journeys seem to take forever and be filled with childish arguments or just long stares out the window. One song always transports me back to the end of a childhood holiday, listening to it now makes me feel nostalgic and sad that I'll never experience that relatively carefree joy of childhood again. It's not a particularly 'happy' song as it's called 'better off alone' but it always makes me remember that dark damp August night sitting in our car. I always remember feeling very low coming home (wishing my holiday wasn't over) and I can still remember the half rain-soaked windscreen and that strange orange street light glow you get here in the UK.

As I got older, going anywhere became harder due to the increasing amounts of equipment I needed and no real friends to visit. Staying home so much meant I had plenty of time for music and when the internet came about I had increasing knowledge of bands. The late nineties for me are signified by my discovery of the *Stereophonics*; a great indie rock band from here in Wales. My sisters were first to introduce me to their CD's of the band and I can remember looking for them on *Yahoo* music. At the time *Yahoo* music allowed you to watch free music videos and listen to some radio stations. I can remember waiting ages on a dial up modem to listen to often poor quality tiny videos of songs like 'Pick a part that's new' and 'Mr Writer'. Whilst in my room I would sing along and get really into the music dissolving away any worries I had.

More recently especially whilst involved with online pool I developed a taste for trance and dance music. Again I suppose I like this sort of instrumental music because it's relaxing and I like to think I'm dancing away in a nightclub! Life seems pretty dull without music and as I'm sitting in front of my computer for hours on end it's great to have a musical diversion. I still sing or hum along quietly to myself as being noisy isn't an option because I now use my computer downstairs. My favourite artists from the trance scene are *Paul Van Dyk, DJ Tiesto, BT* and other various artists found on dance compilation CD's. I'm not really into the loud head banging sort of trance music that you hear a lot of; I like more of the long relaxing tunes that almost sound and feel mystical. I love being transported back into basic thoughts and feelings and into many memories of summers gone by.

As recently as 2009 I got into making my own music via a computer program a friend with DMD recommended. The program has hundreds of instruments in its library and it is tremendous fun making songs. The only downside's being my computers speed and how quickly my hands tire after clicking the various menus and buttons. Another challenging part of music creation is actually coming up with new tunes and melodies. It's not as free as being able to play an actual instrument as it's more like writing music but I find it rewarding and therapeutic. It eats up the time no end but I don't mind that as it's another great way to stop thinking of any worries I may have. I make the music just for fun and sometimes put videos of my tunes on *YouTube*. As the months pass I'm sure I'll make more music and I'll probably change some of my music tastes along the way too.

## Action Duchenne;

Over the last eighteen months I've continued to work voluntarily with *Action Duchenne* producing many more art pieces that help with fundraising; I also campaign to change things here in Wales. I had some sad news in December 2008, when Julia stood down from her position. I had made such friends with her that I was sad she was leaving and worried how my *Action Duchenne* work would continue. Happily we remain good friends and stay in touch on a social networking site. The now vacant position was filled by a lady called Pauline; I had become friends with her on a separate website. I was thrilled she was given the job because she was such a lovely lady and a caring friend who herself had a son with DMD. I'm always amazed by how hard she works and how dedicated she is to the cause. She has become one of my closest friend ever since and in my opinion we work well together.

Pauline was as equally impressed by my art work as Julia was, together we've come up with many projects all aimed at fundraising and awareness. My first project with Pauline as regional development officer was to make a poster and ticket design for an Easter event she was hosting. I painted on the poster a half open egg with goodies inside and the event information was emblazoned on the egg shell itself. The ticket design was along similar lines to the poster but had much less information on it. The event had a fair amount of people turn up and I believe it went down well. I was glad my posters attracted people to our very worthy cause and I had tremendous fun designing all the different elements.

In March Pauline came to visit me at home and I was thrilled to meet my friend in person for the first time. It was a really good meeting and it was so nice breaking up the monotony of my days. Not many friends have actually met me in person so I was really excited when she told me she was coming. She greeted me with a great big hug and we all (including my mother) talked for awhile about all sorts of things. We talked about ideas we had for further fundraising and campaigning and obviously all about DMD. All too soon it was time to say goodbye and I felt really sad as my normal routine would soon take over. Later in the year I visited her house and met her wonderful children, it took a week of working out when to go and how much stuff to take but it is a very happy memory for me.

I've met another wonderful lady who worked for *Action Duchenne* called Victoria. She brought her son (also with DMD), who was most fascinated with my lift and bedroom and asked a lot of questions. I'm always happy to answer questions but I had to be mindful that her son will not yet know all the things I do about DMD. Upsetting him was the very last thing I wanted to do but thankfully I didn't put my 'foot in it'. She also brought her daughter who enjoyed playing with my nephew's toys. Victoria and I talked for awhile and I was fascinated by her Newcastle (mixed with a bit of a Welsh) accent. I'm happy that through *Action Duchenne* I've got to meet new friends and have visitors for the first time in many years. Finally fitting in with a group of people who know and understand where I'm coming from is a lot of comfort to me.

My next 'project' was making a video addressing the delegates at the Welsh Assembly government. I have been in contact with my local AM (assembly member) for the last two years and she thankfully helped setup the 2009 lobby of the Assembly. In my video I asked for a centre of excellence here in Wales, which would be a home to a dedicated team of Duchenne specialists. Currently there isn't a DMD specialist in the whole of Wales and we (sufferers and family) have no where to turn. The only option is to travel hundreds of miles to Newcastle or to London for an (not guaranteed) appointment, for me it may as well be Mars because it's a distance too great. This service should be provided right here in Wales, I am fed up of being swept under the carpet. I ended my video with words along these lines "…all we're asking for is dignity before we die." It was received with a round of applause and also my tribute poem was read out.

I produced many more art related projects after this including a set of awareness posters. These posters gave a new light on what it's like to actually live with this disease and hopefully made people stop and stare. I made a variety of other cards and some new postcard designs. Also I decided to write this very book to raise even more awareness and tell my hopefully interesting story. Finally I've made a painting for auction that features a wonderful scene from right here in Wales. Pauline and I came up with a lot of this in our (legendary in this house) long emails in which we put the world to rights and generally help each other through our respective DMD journeys.

I have continued campaigning by writing to the Welsh Assembly to change local and national care for DMD. I have gone about this by mainly writing emails to the health minister and letting a cross party group hear about the lack of care I receive. The emails have always been answered in the negative, with many promises but little if any action. I feel disappointed after every response as I put a lot effort into writing my emails, often spending hours carefully putting my side of things down and explaining how little we (DMD patients) get in terms of medical care. If you had cancer, cystic fibrosis or diabetes you would expect at least to see a specialist and maybe a few nurses. Receive a bit of treatment maybe but DMD gets none of that here in Wales. Everything is a constant battle.

I feel undervalued like some burden upon the NHS, to be ill and forgotten about is an awful feeling. It is little wonder why many Muscular Dystrophy patients (it's a condition wide problem) suffer from depression and other mental illnesses. This drives me on to get things changed for not only me but the many children coming into an even poorer adult care situation. Although I can't do it on my own, we need more people to be writing letters and showing politicians how dire things are in Wales and the UK. It can't be fair that lads and a small amount of ladies with DMD, a disease we are born with and didn't choose get almost zero health care! Save the odd time we need emergency medical admissions because of a lack of monitoring. This unfairness has got to end.

Another unexpected part of working with *Action Duchenne* has been providing support for others going through this disease namely the parents. Having been through most of the stressful parts of Duchenne, I offer my advice as to what my family did in certain situations that commonly arise with DMD. If there's an issue raised about adaptations, I would say how my bedroom had been altered and how my house was altered. Practical advice is much easier to give than say emotional advice but my positive attitude always helps me get through. I always try to be sympathetic and caring but sometimes you just need to agree with how bad things are. In those situations I just offer my hugs (virtual as I talk to most people online) and am there just to understand. We have to be there for each other!

My relationship with other older guys living with DMD is mostly very good as we share a common feeling of just getting on with life. We don't want to really talk about DMD as most of us aren't desperately clinging on to get a potential cure. While it would be nice to get a cure, we aren't deluded by what science is coming up with at the moment. A viable treatment to slow DMD down is a more realistic option but we/I realise that it's a few years away. Time is not something we have a lot of so I suppose we just try to live as much of a life as we can before the inevitable happens. That's not to stay we always see eye to eye on everything. Sometimes I have felt like 'letting the team down' when I have a negative day but as we all experience DMD differently, we can't be expected to feel the same things. I see us as a band of brothers and some sisters all going through our personal battles with DMD but it always hurts when we lose someone dear to us with whom we became friends.

## Family:

A lovely new addition to the family has been my lovely niece Nia. She was born in 2008 and has been a joy ever since then. I loved watching her grow from a beautiful baby into a cheeky giggling toddler. I have fond memories of her pinching my foot blanket and tickling my feet. I'm always amazed how quickly babies grow and how quickly things are learnt. She can say all the usual things like 'mammy', 'daddy', 'nana', 'gran-dad' etc, and has even learnt to say her brother's name 'Iwan'. Lately she has learned many words and comes out with new things all the time; she says 'Sian' and my name in her very cute little voice. I love listening to her giggles and when she sings songs with her mum. All this melts my heart and if I've had a bad day just one happy thought of Nia makes me feel a lot better. If I ever had children of my own I'd want them to be just like Nia and Iwan, full of life, cheeky, cute and independent.

Iwan has continued to grow up reaching the age of four. It's been great watching him transitioning from learning to talk right up to his now bilingual speech. His mother wanted her children to be taught the language of Welsh; it has really made a come back here in Wales. Iwan can tell us all the colours in Welsh and have quite a good conversation with his mother. Sadly I never really picked it up but I do know a few words and listen to some Welsh music. He's quite an inquisitive lad, asking me lots of questions about the computer games I play. For instance he wanted to know if my flight simulator control panel was a car's dashboard, he was most fascinated when I showed him an aeroplane flying. It's great to see him bounding into our house playing with a stash of toys we have in a nook between the television and dresser. His newest fad is pulling the seats off our sofa pretending to make slides and cars out of them. I hope I continue seeing Iwan and Nia growing up just to see their smiles and carefree joy.

Ceri my brother in law (Emma's husband) is a fantastic guy. When he first came into the family I can remember how tall and how shy he was, my uncle Alan used to tease him something chronic. The poor guy's face would go bright red but he has since built up a laid back nature just like Emma. We always recall the time he was feeding me a ham sandwich and my throat decided to choke, but very calmly he helped me pull out the offending piece of meat. Subsequently he has vowed never to feed me ham sandwiches ever again! We all have a laugh about this still, but true to his word he never ever put ham near me again. I was really happy when he asked Emma to marry him; he is absolutely perfect for my sister and a fabulous father to Iwan and Nia. It's always nice to see him when he pops over our house with the children or if he needs to borrow tools from my fathers shed. His sense of humour is great too always joking to Sian about anything she may have done. We tease each other about our thinning hair which is really funny. He's also very helpful taking my parents out when they need a lift and always offering to lend a hand.

My relationship with my eldest sister Emma is really good even though she's not living at home anymore. On the plus side she only moved few hundred yards away. I see her when she picks up the children or comes to visit on the weekends. We don't say loads to each other, just enough to get by, I speak far more to her on a social network site; which makes our mother laugh. Emma's always been encouraging, whether it's cheering me up or explaining something to me. For example when it looked like I would need a feeding tube, she showed me a similar type some of her pupils were using at her job. One memory we always laugh and reminisce over was time a hot baked bean fell on my foot! She was busily preparing a meal and being a 'curious George' I just had to go look what she was doing. I had gotten too near the stove when a stray bean dropped and landed on my foot, I hobbled into the next room (I could walk back then) and said lots of garbled pained nonsense. We got the bean off eventually but I still have a reminder on my foot. We always laugh over that bean! Emma's a great sister always kind and cheerful and caring. She even bought me legwarmers this winter when I mentioned them.

Sian and I have always had the typical brother and sister relationship. We would argue white is black and water was vinegar. Strangely we have always had similar taste in music, we would (and still) both say 'I like that' in unison when I had a cassette, CD or when listening to the radio. It was good to have that kind of childhood relationship as it made us both feel totally 'normal', there was no DMD when we listened to music or watched our favourite programmes on television. As we both grew older we each had our own problems, Sian with her reading and me with the growing progression of Duchenne. We would still have the odd argument but we grew closer; when our parents went out we would have a light hearted chat about music, food and the family dog. When she left to go to university it was like I was losing a friend but only briefly as she would visit often. It was good to see her move back home after her degree in textiles was over, finding various jobs and going out with her friends. It's fun to hear about all her adventures 'out with the girls' around our locale. Sort of like a connection to the outside world for me. Now we still have our chats but mainly about relationships, Duchenne and pretty much life in general. Sian's an out going girl with lots of laughs and plenty of stories to tell.

My relationship with my father is very good but like every father and son we often disagree on the odd thing. As a child he would take me swimming and guide my horse when I used to ride all those years ago. I used to accompany him to an allotment he used to own, taking our dog there for company. While he dug away planting seeds and pointing out different wildlife to me, I would lay on an old leather seat watching the sky fly by talking to my dog. Getting thirsty around noon I would follow him to a wonderfully smelling shed with an ancient kettle and we all had tea or I just had milk. I remember summers driving my wheelchair next to my father down a path called the 'Taf Trail' spotting all the types of trees. We collected blackberries and sped through patches of flying midges. I am always grateful for the time he said he was happy with whatever I wanted to do. I still talk to him about my day, how my art is going, how my campaigning letters are being received and asking lots of science questions. I sometimes help him out drawing designs for a few of his work projects and searching for websites on the internet. If my mother goes out he'll look after me and we'll watch action movies and have a laugh. If I ever need anything built my father's always there to make something, he fashioned my head rest, made me a drink holder and even replaced my table top to name but a few. If we do have any disagreements they are quickly forgotten and we move on in our usual jovial way.

My mother is a mum first and a fantastic carer second and we are really close. I cannot tell you how grateful I am for all she has done and continues to do. It must have been tough at diagnosis knowing her son was extremely ill and dealing with all the other misinformed parents who thought I was a 'contagious' kid. I always remember her as being strong and loving throughout my childhood and now into my adulthood. She has always backed me up when things piled on me, instilling a 'get up and go' mentality that continues to drive me. We've always tried to attack things positively and if I just need a hug or reassurance she's right there behind me. For instance when my teacher in secondary school claimed I was 'possessive' over a carer, my mother told him how out of character that sounded and that was the end of that. Other great memories I have revolve around the times we had to visit the other side of my village when I was a child, the dentist and GP are all there so this was quite regular. We would always pop in to the chip shop and sit nearby watching the world go past. Now though my care needs have 'exploded' so we are stuck at home a lot more, everyday my mother suctions my chest and dresses me and takes me to toilet and feeds me and looks after the things everyday mothers do. As you can imagine this is very tiring for her and sometimes understandably late at night we may have an argument; but they are quickly forgotten about. My mother is great, always supporting and I frequently tell her 'I love you Mam' while she's helping me out, she really is a special lady.

Other members of my family often come to visit at various times of the month. My Uncle Alan and Cousin Sean pop in after work on the odd occasion. Bringing with them stories of the industrial estate they work at. Sean tells me about all the cars he's seen while repairing them. I learn loads about spark plugs, timing belts, ignition coils and body work repairs. I'm quite interested in engines especially now that I'm into Formula one. All those intricate parts working together in balance is amazing if you think about it. I think older cars have more charm than these newer 'bubble' cars as I call them. Uncle Alan is a welder which is really hard work and challenging. I'm fascinated in how welding works; it's like gluing metal together but using more metal as the 'adhesive'. Alan tells me what projects he's been doing or how busy the workshop is; this varies week by week. It's good to hear all the stories of my extended family too, as generally I don't go anywhere. My grand parents visit rarely but they will often ring up to check how everyone is. If they've cooked something for us they'll let us know too, they make apple tarts and corned beef pasties for all the family. Sadly I can't eat any of it but that is not the point and I think it's a wonderful gesture considering how frail they are.

## The Future:

Well you've made it to the final section of my book and for me it's time to look ahead to the future. I'm increasingly realising that my time is fast running out. Recently I received a less than positive prognosis; my geneticist told me that the time between a treatment being available for me and me being able to receive it looks too great. Considering there could be a treatment within the next two to three years, effectively I've been given less than that to live. I don't really know how to take this news except that as usual I have to continue ploughing on fighting this disease. I'm obviously upset by the thought of an early death and as I'm writing this my eyes are filling with tears. I've got to be strong and continue fighting for better care for all the boys who are starting or ending their individual fights with Duchenne. I've also got to prepare what happens after the 'big' sleep but I'm not sure what to do.

The geneticist has recommended I write a will and got me in contact with a palliative care doctor. I have since started writing a will but it's so difficult wondering what to do. Originally I wanted an 'over the top' coffin but have since realised that A) I can't look at it for obvious reasons and B) I don't think it is respectful to our creator God. Now I want something more toned down and fit for purpose in a dark wood. I'd like my pocket watch collection to be auctioned and the proceeds to go to *Action Duchenne*. I've even written out something I want read at my funeral just as my final goodbye. I'm hoping that this book will help raise more awareness. Also most of the money it raises through royalties will go straight to *Action Duchenne*. Even if I can't stop DMD in my lifetime I want to continue helping even after I'm gone.

I met the palliative care doctor a few months ago and the meeting seemed to go well. The doctor just basically outlined what she did and what they could do to help me. If I'm ever stuck in hospital needing equipment or need help to leave, they are just a phone call away with advice and are experts in getting people the care they need at home. Sadly as I don't go into hospital very much it seemed there was little else they could offer me. When they asked if there was anything I needed, I was unsure because I thought they were going to be offering me more. I didn't know so I said 'not that I can think of,' at that point she had to rush off after only half an hour. She left us for some reason in the 'capable hands' of a dietician who works on her floor. I have yet to hear from this dietician but she has to come weigh me soon anyway. Other than that if I want them I'll need to give them a ring. Frankly I feel a bit abandoned.

On a more general Duchenne note I'm hoping the future brings a viable treatment that's much better than the current stop gap measure of steroids. They aren't ideal causing many side effects such as weight gain, behavioural imbalances, osteoporosis, a 'moon' face (rounded by the medication) and height deficiencies. They cause other problems with the immune system (weakening it), so that constant monitoring is needed. If the child/young adult is unwell with a cold or flu symptoms an increased covering dose of steroids is required to help them overcome it. In some cases steroids are not appropriate for every person with DMD. In my case I missed the whole steroid 'boat' a long time ago. I have great hope that a replacement treatment can be found with much fewer side effects and accessible to every DMD patient. The main stumbling block is time and obviously the funding required but these can be and will be bypassed.

I hope within a decade the eventual cure will come at least to a point where DMD people can lead practically 'normal' lives. I can't predict the future so all I can do is give my informed opinion but I really hope the days of ventilators and feeding tubes are going to end. There are lots of clinical trials in progress all over the world and the horizon for DMD looks a lot brighter. It still hurts that so many more boys and some girls will die before these treatments come onto the market. It really is a race against time and I find it very ironic that I'm really fascinated by watches and chronology. Every few weeks I hear of another DMD patient dying and it tears and rips at me every time. The overwhelming feeling of sadness I always get reminds me that my time is short; I just hate that feeling knowing I could be next, I'm worried I'll become another 'statistic'. The general public usually have very little knowledge of all these deaths but as well as funding and time DMD needs far more general awareness.

I have one further ambition before I die and that is to produce my best piece of art. I can see my talents increasing every year so I want to leave a most impressive painting as a legacy. I really enjoy producing paintings, sketching out landscapes and finally applying the digital oil paint I love working with. One of my best has been **Aurora Borealis** (found in a previous section) it has got so many thousand views on *DeviantArt* that I'm really overwhelmed. I still feel there is more to come from me now that I've got back to painting in a more direct way. I'm not sure if it'll come as a landscape of as a portrait but I'm positive I'll have fun along the way. I always wonder if my work will hang in a gallery one day, with many visitors peering at the work I did on a painting program using an old fashioned 'mouse'. I often have dreams of my work selling for millions but common sense takes over and I think 'nah, that'll never happen' but in case it does as ever the proceeds should go to Action Duchenne.

Finally I want to close this book on a message of hope inspired by my belief in God. The Holy Bible assures us that death is not the end of things. If we obey God he will give us the greatest gift that being an immortal spiritual life in something called the millennial kingdom. Every one (just or unjust) will get resurrected in at least one of two such resurrections (find out more in the book of Revelation). If found 'just' we will be welcomed into this new spiritual life with new bodies. At that time there'll be no DMD, no war, no hatred, no famine and Jesus will return as our king. This wonderful gift can only be accessed if you walk in the ways of God and believe that Jesus has taken our sins away through his tragic death nailed to the cross. Its not easy being a Christian but it sure is worth it to get a second chance at a perfect life.

Even if you have never heard of or studied Jesus and the Holy Bible you will get a chance during the second resurrection. Thus we can welcome loads of our family members into a new perfect life too!

Hope of this wonderful future after we die has helped me on the very difficult days when I feel alone and depressed. An excellent way of describing this current life in relation to the next is to think of it as a seed, all our trials and tribulations and how we fight them are 'growing' this seed. When we reach that second life the hopefully fully grown seed will be our new 'glorified' body waiting for us. Here is a better description found in the Holy Bible, Romans Chapter eight Verse eighteen 'For I reckon that the sufferings of this present time are not worthy to be compared with the glory which shall be revealed in us'. Our current tough lives are just a test so with that attitude in mind I find things just a little bit easier to handle.

By no means does this mean that our lives are easy or our needs are any less important. The Holy Bible tells us to care for our fellow man and in this current world you don't see a lot of care around. It's always pleasing to see acts of kindness in the news and not the usual awfulness we see. It's even more vital that everyone becomes more loving and caring so that many more of us can reach the millennial kingdom together. I know many who don't share my views but it really will be a fabulous gift when the time comes. In closing I wish every one of my friends and family and to everyone else who reads this book all the best in your lives and pursuits. Together we'll beat Duchenne Muscular Dystrophy once and for all.

# *Latest Update Chapter*

As this book chronicles the first twenty five years of my life, I won't be going through every individual year since publishing because I want to be faithful to that. Its been five years since publishing and six years since I finished the actual writing, so I thought I'd do an update in case people were curious about my life since then.

## My Life Currently:

A lot has happened over the last few years with my condition, especially in one particular area - that being sleeping times as I rarely get to sleep before four in the morning! It takes two hours of suctioning and bed time preparation before I can drift off. Starting earlier isn't really an option given the fact that I finish the last meal of the day by twelve thirty in the early hours. Obviously I need to let that digest a bit and there's another medication to take and during this time I *Skype* one of my dear friends. So by one thirty to two in the morning I start this gruelling bed time procedure. It impacts on my mother the most because of her tiredness and fatigue which always makes me feel sad. The poor woman only gets four hours sleep but some nights we do get to bed earlier. Sometimes my chest won't be full of secretions meaning that we get to bed by three in the morning.

After a tracheotomy tube change and when my suction machine is at peak efficiency this can happen. I always thank God when this occurs because I know He is involved in my life.

Shortly after writing six years ago I met another lady who I briefly dated and amazingly for me she often visited me at home. We watched *YouTube* videos and she played the guitar which I really enjoyed. Sadly I seem expert at ruining my relationships and I said things I really regret and did things I regret especially becoming obsessed with unsavoury things that spoiled her trust. I don't think we were really compatible and I rushed in to a relationship for selfish desires. I'm still friends with her which I'm grateful for but I hope I'm not the same kind of man now because I want to be a gentleman. DMD and relationships don't always mix but there are success stories out there and maybe I'll find the right lady to complete me one day.

As Duchenne's progresses I continue to get weaker and here is a small list of changes. Firstly my hands are greatly weakened and solely using a regular mini optical mouse is very tiring. I've been blessed with a new gadget called a *Tobii PCEYE GO* that tracks my eyes to move the cursor around the screen and allows me to click with blinks. I use this in conjunction with the aforementioned mouse. Secondly my neck muscles are really struggling, it has become a real difficulty keeping my head up. My ingenious father has found a solution using a sweatband attached to my headrest which I find very useful. Thirdly I've noticed my voice becoming quieter and I'm needing to repeat myself more often which is highly frustrating.

It becomes most apparent when travelling to medical appointments in our van because no matter how much I try to raise my voice my parents struggle to hear me. Although that has more to do with my noisy van which is much quieter now after a recent repair. Fourthly my ventilator use has increased to twenty one to twenty two hours on a bad day. The last cold I had saw it get near twenty four hours but that's to be expected. I used roughly five hundred suction catheters that week - to put it into perspective I usually use roughly two hundred a week. Fifthly my swallowing very slowly declines but pureed food still keeps me going and a company called *Wiltshire Farm Foods* helps take the load off my parents with their range of pre-packaged pureed meals. Duchenne Muscular Dystrophy is such a relentless disease but you definitely see how resilient this physical body can be and sadly how fragile life really is.

A related issue surrounding my life with this all encompassing condition is that of my drinking straw. As most people using a nasal ventilator mask know, any air leakages can blow a straw away from the mouth quite easily. It's frustrating asking for it to be moved back into place and I'm sure it frustrates my caregivers. Sometimes when talking on *Skype* to one of my best friends she feels my pain when the straw decides it wants to "fly" around. She is several thousand miles away and wishes she could flick that straw back to me. Thankfully that has been rectified with something called a straw clip which I found online. It was recommended to me by Carl mentioned a few chapters ago as he understood the issue I was going through. I wanted to thank him personally but I sadly never got the chance because he recently died.

A twenty eight year old shining light in the world of Duchenne's taken to soon. It hit me really hard, I was numb all day especially reading everyone's comments and tributes. Later I cried while my parents were cooking in the other room, the tears just flowed along with throat constricting near silent sobs. You never get used to death - it hurts losing friends but I have great hope of seeing them again.

Moving onto my chest, like any condition I can have good days or bad and this is definitely true with my lungs. On good days I may have just one or two periods of suction using ten catheters per period give or take a few. On a bad day I could have five or more periods of suctioning which is physically exhausting and frustrating as each session takes forty minutes to an hour and a half! My mother gets very tired and sometimes arguments ensue which is totally understandable although we both regret it later and say sorry. You have to get into forgiving attitudes with DMD. Also on bad days transfers from wheelchair to bed and from chair to bathroom are fraught with anxiety and sometimes pain.

It's hard work when nearly every transfer makes me feel like coughing my ineffective coughs and it sometimes gets to me psychologically too. My chest feels like a bag of nails as I describe it and breathing just through my nose is difficult. I don't use my ventilator when transferring so I feel like I'm in an ever tightening strait jacket constricting my lungs and giving me a headache. I'm gasping when the procedure is done but prayers get me through it. Also all this movement stirs up my chest starting up the familiar rattle that causes more anxiety.

When that happens I'm calling my mother to take me back to the suction machine and those short moments seem like ages when you can't breathe. Eventually I may need to wear my ventilator during these transfers but hopefully not too soon.

It's difficult watching your body continually failing and weakening every week, every month and every year. Most of the time I try not to dwell on it or give it much thought but in a small way, like grief, it hits you every so often. I'll admit that I miss eating regular food especially bread, pastry, anything crunchy, eating out and the British favourite - fish and chips. It's difficult watching others eat but I generally don't mind because I don't want to be miserable all day. Also very hard to take is not being able to give a hug to anyone (which may have been mentioned earlier). It has become quite apparent when conversing with friends or when the little children from my family are here. I long to pick up the kids, play games and generally do constructive things with them. That's a tough thing to deal with.

It occurred to me that it would be interesting to mention what being totally dependent on others is like. If a crease is left in the cover my arms rest on for bed, then several hours later it feels like a knife is sticking in me. Obviously I ask for such creases to be removed which can seem pedantic to my parents but immobility means I could deal with increasing amounts of pain if it isn't done. Another example is my back which can become very painful because of scoliosis and the placement of my shirt or hoisting sling. I don't always at first let my caregivers know about it because of the workload they are under from a whole lot of scratching, moving of arms, sorting my wheelchair out, wiping my eyes, often suctioning, correction of my computer's position and various other things that go on. I really don't like to irritate them especially as tempers could flare from sleep deprivation and a high workload. I have to pick the least stressful time to ask and some slight corrections of my shirt or sling can help greatly, I must balance this against the extreme pain because I can't stay like that. Who could? This kind of balancing act is necessary because keeping a happy home is paramount alongside personal comfort.

Being dependent on someone for absolutely everything is challenging and a multi-complex thing. There's sometimes worries and concerns that a sudden mishap might happen stranding me without help. I can briefly think, "What if a caregiver gets hurt and I'm off my ventilator and my chest fills with mucus?" That kind of thought used to be terrifying to me and that's where faith has really helped me because I can take my worries to a Higher Power and relax. Even so, I'm human and still worries can creep in, it can be stressful when those moments arrive. It can be most acute when I do have a full chest and seemingly minutes or seconds until breathing becomes impossible - at that time it's frantic. I rush my mother who, like superwoman, gets me to the suction machine and the muck is removed and thoughts of how close I just came to death occasionally surface. How long will I keep making it to the suction machine in the nick of time? It's not my place to answer but it sure makes one think. An excellent description from the parents' point of view is given by my friend Dave, who is a parent of a lad with DMD his blog is here; *http://www.davidlclick.com/blog/like-an-old-married-couple* - check it out.

Finally I want to briefly mention how centrally important to my life faith has been. I've grown from my first tentative steps in faith into knowing a precious amount about the Holy Bible. I won't try converting anyone because it's for each and everyone of us to make our personal decision. I've met and fellowshipped with some absolutely wonderful people who are very dear to me. Unless you have experienced God's influence in your life you'll never know the joy of answered prayers. I've had amazing personal interventions and have seen God help others in His Church. I remember that I was once having trouble with my suction machine it, wouldn't suction me with the correct power. My chest was suffering badly and I felt really tired.

I prayed about it and over the course of six months God intervened by getting me on my backup machine which helped. However the main suction machine still wasn't right no matter what the local nurses tried. I was getting desperate and down to my last option of contacting my respiratory consultant. Before that appointment, one morning out of the blue my mother had a phone call from the nurses that others had had this problem and miraculously they figured out the issue. A simple gasket was worn out, it was changed and the machine worked! I realize you could deny this but I know it was God sorting everything out for me behind the scenes. God seldom works as you would expect and always in His time frame. Finally I believe He will heal me either through death (hard to understand but I know what I mean) or in this life.

## Death and Duchenne:

A difficult but I feel necessary part of DMD is the subject of death. Whether you're a parent who has anticipatory grief knowing their child will die, or someone living with this condition watching their friends die from it, death certainly affects us all. I have lost a number of friends and acquaintances over these last few years and it's very hard because I invariably end up thinking of my own mortality. DMD cruelly strikes down those who look well on the outside but their insides are being battered. Even though I have great hope and have faith death still hurts and is difficult to face. I really hope my final moments if death does pounce on me early will be relatively quick and painless. On my darkest and most morose days I look forward to a rest in the grave. When my chest is really rough and on days of extreme discomfort and pain I just want to have some relief. That's not to say I want euthanasia because I don't believe in killing myself. I do however ask God for relief in whatever way He knows I need. Usually the next day I feel brighter and I'm able to positively move on.

This very book is dedicated to my friend Sam who died five years ago. After his death I was numb for days. It hit hard because he lived near and even though we could never meet we had a great connection as friends on the internet. His mother was very kind recently saying that I've helped her through her grief. If I can help I will, with God's guidance leading me of course, because I'm no specialist on grief. I've been in contact with a few mothers who have lost their children to this terrible condition. I see that grief doesn't really have stages it's all emotions thrown together and time is rarely a healer. Unless you have hope for the future about what happens after death it all seems hopeless. These families do continue their lives taking their memories everywhere they go and some heroically keep on helping those families still facing DMD with their children. I feel that any contribution I make to their plight is very small indeed.

I know of at least eight personal friends who died because of DMD or things related to the condition. I lost two this year alone and know of many others who have succumbed to this deadly disease. It does feel like a thousand cuts sometimes because social media has informed me of so much death. Don't get me wrong social media is vital to the Duchenne's community but it has downsides too. It will be so good when this disease no longer claims lives and no child learns to walk only for it to be cruelly snatched away. That day will come, if you're suffering with the loss of a child hold onto any hope you can find and if I could, I'd hug you. If you have got DMD and are facing death daily try not to fear - because death is like sleeping, which is comforting. Focus on what you can do on a day to day basis and do what you need to find relief when that time comes.

That brings me to an interesting question about my faith that you may be wondering about especially regarding these deaths, that being "why would God allow anyone to have suffered DMD in the first place, if He is all powerful?" I remember thinking before God started using me, "what is the point of life if I'm going to die young". Reading through the *Hitchhikers Guide to the Galaxy* I came across the idea of the meaning of life, I metaphorically ate the book only to get the silly answer 42. It ignited a curiosity into that subject and God answered that, because basically He is reproducing Himself through mankind. Every human has a potential within this great plan and that includes those with DMD.

Back to the main question and why would God allow DMD into this world? First of all God created Spiritual laws but crucially also physical laws of health whose transgression result in sickness and illness. Now it's not necessarily something deliberately done wrong, it could be a bacteria or something else even genetic that made you ill. Nevertheless these health laws have been transgressed. Sadly many think that God deliberately gives us DMD but it's not His fault at all, it's simply the breaking of these health laws. This has been neglected by the world and is never really taught by mankind's religions or doctors.

You might think "surely God could quickly end this suffering especially as His Son's amazing sacrifices have taken the penalties of transgression away?" There's something far bigger going on and it has everything to do with God reproducing Himself. God wants everyone to be like Him eventually and to bring about repentance for all mankind. Repentance means to turn, and what we must turn from is our own human ways which have led to this present suffering world. However it also means that we must turn to God, His Ways and a whole lot more.

At this time God is not bringing all to repentance but in a specific time order of His choosing. Those chosen now are in training for an important future job helping God to fulfil His plan. For the billions of as yet uncalled in this world God has adopted a "hand's off" policy. Mankind is learning the lesson of aversion therapy so that we become so thoroughly sick of this world of appalling depravity and sickness that we never want to repeat these mistakes ever again. This is what truly will bring about mass repentance and once we learn our lesson all suffering and sickness will be eradicated. There certainly will be life after death and there's tremendous hope ahead.

## Family changes:

Moving from death to life now as we have new arrivals in the family. Firstly my sister Sian got married in 2013 to a wonderfully kind and caring man called Mathew. He currently works as a theatre nurse and is a hard worker. Sian is a carrier of DMD so trying for children would always be difficult. She went through an uncomfortable process called IVF specifically PGD (pre-implantation growth diagnosis). After one failed attempt there was success and excitingly she was pregnant. During their initial scans the consultant sat Sian and Mat down and said there were two bits of good news. The new parents thinking that their baby was doubly blessed hadn't realized the consultant meant twins! To say they were shocked was an understatement but how wonderful, I thought!

She gave birth via caesarean section in November 2014 and had two beautiful girls who were named Eira Mai (pronounced A-Ra, My) and Meagan Louise. Sadly they were born premature by six weeks because Sian was ill. Thankfully they were relatively healthy and after a few weeks in the special care baby unit they came home. Sian still lives nearby but not next door like she had previously. The babies continue to grow and develop albeit slightly behind due to their prematurity. They are just over a year old now and I love them to bits. I have been fascinated by twins ever since they were born and every time I hear about twins I really take notice. I've seen a few television programmes on twins and I'm fascinated by mirror twins. For instance they will have opposite handedness i.e. left handed for one, right handed for the other. So far our twins are doing this but it's very early days to be certain, it's all extremely exciting. As mentioned earlier I miss being able to hold the twins and interact with them, there's just a deep yearning to be able to do things although I try not dwelling on that.

Now we come to Emma and her family. Her husband Ceri works for a national supermarket chain helping find new locations for stores and of course Emma is still a special needs teacher. Iwan her eldest child is ten would you believe and is football obsessed - he trains and plays too. It's amazing how much he can eat but that's to be expected when you run around a lot. He loves our satellite television and is into *XBOX* gaming. Nia is seven which is astounding as you wonder where the time goes. She loves pink and is our little princess, she's a very kind, extremely outgoing and caring girl who can be a tomboy sometimes too. Also she's really into the stage, going nearly weekly to *Stagecoach* who train her with drama, singing and dancing and has appeared locally in a nearby theatre. Both are fond of their uncle but especially Nia.

Nia has a habit of staring intently at me lost in her thoughts, my mother looks at me and says "there will be questions" and usually her mother will get them. Questions like "why couldn't I walk?" and many others that I can't think of off the top of my head. One particularly funny memory I have was when she drew a picture of me with these strange appendages surrounding my legs. She explained that these were Uncle Ian's working legs, my immediate reaction was "aww that's sweet, love her" - she really cares about me. Her mother was shocked and was thankful that I was quite laid back about it all. I think Nia really wants me to interact with her, play and draw etc. I definitely wish I could. For now at least she's content to talk with me and watch me do some art on my computer, sometimes joining in. When she draws sometimes she asks me what to draw and what colours to use etc. She recently saw a television programme with soldiers in prosthetics and wondered if that would help me, to which her mother said "no". She must be constantly thinking about how to help me which definitely makes me say "aww".

My parents are still doing relatively well although they have both had  minor surgeries. When my mother went in for hers my father looked after me which was difficult because my mother is the main caregiver. We managed pretty well and worked together as best as possible. My poor father had a long recovery after his operation but now is doing well again. All their grandchildren love them very dearly especially the newest additions, who enjoy being held by them. They look after Nia and Iwan for usually three nights weekly during term time and they see the twins quite often too. My father has recently retired from being a university professor but has thrown himself into helping my mother care for me. He has been on a few cooking courses and his lemon drizzle cakes and fruitcakes are very nice but sadly I can't eat those because of my swallowing issues. However I can eat his soup so long as it's blended, I really enjoy his leek and potato creation. I'm extremely grateful for the superb care and love that my parents give me.

## Updating DMD information:

One thing I've noticed more and more recently is that the whole story on DMD is not being told correctly. Too often in literature aimed at raising awareness you see statements saying that only boys get this condition. That's not entirely correct because in rare cases girls can get this condition through some pretty strange genetic interactions. There are actually types of carriers who are severely manifesting, there are other manifesting carriers with lesser symptoms and unaffected carriers. Sometimes DMD seemingly happens spontaneously but I won't debate that here because of the complexity. A better way to write the information is to say it primarily affects boys and in rare cases girls. I think those with awareness in mind should try to cover the whole devastating story but I'm not criticizing, just suggesting a more holistic approach. I'm friends with a few severely manifesting carriers so I've seen how left out they can feel, no one should be invisible like they sometimes are.

New understanding about what causes DMD may be on the horizon because a lot of research is being done.

Amazingly I know that a few treatments are nearly available, with governments around the world approving them. There are a few caveats however, it will help a small percentage only and only those who can still walk. One particular drug could help up to thirteen percent of those affected. In reality it'll be fewer based on this ambulation requirement which strikes me as extremely unfair. I can see why it's being done because it was tested on ambulatory candidates and there are no ways currently of testing non-ambulatory trial participants.

If a drug is approved it should be available to all who could benefit regardless of ambulation. Just because you can't walk doesn't mean your life is over, preserving breathing and heart function could still offer benefits and who knows, maybe a slight improvement in the overall condition might ensue. How can it be known that the non-ambulatory will benefit if they are never given the chance. Eventually the researchers may include the non ambulatory but how many must die before then? Withholding it now creates a kind of apartheid where DMD is a death sentence once you're off your feet. I'm not saying I'm relying on scientists to heal me because I believe that is God's department. I'm just pointing out an unfair situation in potential treatments that could give those with DMD some much needed help.

### Art and writing updated:

Over the last few years I've continued doing my digital art, I got heavily into jewellery design producing digital images of rings, earrings and pendants. I've done tens and tens of them but only had three pieces made into reality, two pendants and a ring. One pendant I designed as a wedding gift for my sister Sian, it depicted "falling" maple leaves all in silver with two specific leaves having many cubic zirconium stones crammed in. It looked wonderful on my sister during her special day. I was thrilled with how the other pendant turned out it looked like a half moon on a dark blue night all in enamel with a gold circular surround. There were various other golden parts and seven diamonds included in the piece. The ring depicts a starry night, it is a gold ring coated in black enamel with a few diamonds dotted all around. I really like how all of my real jewellery pieces turned out.

Recently I've moved on from jewellery to other things because I never like staying in one area too long. It was also in small part due to the disappointment of not actually being able to make what I was designing. I was getting a deep subconscious yearning to create jewellery for real. I've got some semi-precious stones here that I use as a reference and I'd love to make something with them. It's not great to feel so unfulfilled as an artist so I do far less jewellery designing now. On the positive side I did enter two jewellery competitions over the last two years. It was a hugely fun and challenging time designing and printing the jewellery images and getting them sent off. Sadly I didn't win for all that effort but I'm under no illusions about my designing abilities.

Now I'm into pixel art after a friend also living with DMD recommended it to me. I've had an interest in all things miniature for awhile so to make my own tiny art in a digital format is rewarding. I use a free basic program called *Paint.NET* to make my pixel art. I create 100 square pixel canvases or 200 square pixel canvases and zoom in to make the images one pixel at a time. The only downside is how do I get these tiny images on products available for sale on the internet? The solution was to stitch the images together in a sort of digital patchwork quilt if you will. I fill a 2000 square pixel canvas with many 200 square pixel images and these are particularly effective as phone covers. By the way I'm no longer selling art on *DeviantArt* but I'm using *Redbubble.com* now. You can view my profile here at *http://www.redbubble.com/people/thebigg2005* - please check it out.

A while ago I wanted to improve my digital art skills especially with my art program called *Corel Painter*. I found a few tutorials on *YouTube* and I learned more about fully using *Corel Painter*. I tried new styles of painting including impressionism and purely digital techniques. I enjoyed making an impressionistic image of a windmill on a riverside in bright bold colours, which was well received. It really helps to see what other artists do, it can really spark your interest and give you ideas. So the internet continues to improve as a resource for artists and as a medium for sales. If you're an artist check out *Corel Painter* tutorials or any art tutorials on *YouTube*, even if you're not an artist you can definitely buy loads of beautiful things online.

Moving on to my writing now which has had its ups and down. I wrote an ebook a few years back which collates all my poetry into a coherent collection. It has descriptions detailing why I wrote them and what each poem meant to me and was called *Poetic Diversions*. Which you can find here; *https://www.smashwords.com*

*/books/view/206857* - I hope you really enjoy reading it. I also occasionally write a blog all about this very book and my experiences living with DMD. You can view this here; *http://inspiredlifebook.blogspot.co.uk/* - it is definitely a worthwhile read. My poetry writing has been very sparse since I wrote *Poetic Diversions* but recently I had inspiration. I came up with an intense poem called *DMD Reality*, which was about what I was feeling on a bad day and this is what I'll end this section with.

The bright shiny day beckons,
Oh what to do, a world of opportunity awaits I reckon,
But no, my back decides to hurt whichever way I sit,
Painkillers would only mask the hit,
It's positioning, you see,
I have Duchenne Muscular Dystro-phy,
What a rotter and a plotter,
Plotting my daily destruction, potentially mere minutes from death at any given time,
No one knows their time,
Not even me with DMD,
It could be the heart or respiratory failure,
I'm older you see, it could be any number of things in the pail, yea,
I had palpitations - a crazy flutter in heart rhythm,
Tens of uncontrollable fast beats, is this it?....
...........

...............
No, still here, have no fear,
A relief but also not, if you know what I mean,
I'm still imprisoned you see, trapped in ever decreasing circles,

Trapped in my own body,
No exercise time, recess, lunch or free periods to escape this cell, it's 24/7,
I'm going through the rain now, but sunshine follows the storm,
There remains hope, truth and a shining brilliant future of freedom will be the norm.

## What would it be like;

If you have ever seen the movie *The Theory of Everything* you will remember the scene where the lead actor gets up out of his wheelchair and walks in a vision. His body corrects itself, he picks up a pen and hands it back to an audience member and all this was very surreal. I know of another with DMD who wrote about a day with his walking restored. For the last few years I've been meditating on this very topic wondering what it would be like to be cured. Some might think that this would be torture but actually it offers hope and gets me through tough times. The only downside is immediately afterwards when I can't do what I envisioned and occasionally a pang of disappointment briefly washes over me. I want to write what I think may happen in the days and weeks following a cure.

During my daydreams I usually start waking up in my bed with my ventilator on. Suddenly I fling my arms in the air and look in wonder at my now moving hands and fingers. Then I slide my legs out from under the covers and quietly stagger to my feet holding my nearby wheelchair for support. I'm still wearing my ventilator mask so I carefully prise it off making sure to cover the tubing. This will prevent the alarm sounding, while covering the pipe I go over to my ventilator and switch it off muting the alarm every time it sounds. Hopefully my parents haven't noticed this procedure because I'm itching to surprise them! Whilst doing all this I'd be thanking God and just beaming with a huge smile then I'd put on some underwear and jogging bottoms. They are special wheelchair joggers so I would imagine having to wrestle to keep them on which would be humorous no doubt.

How liberating it will be to breathe on my own without feeling like a gasping rasping man. Deep lungfuls of air will feel fantastic and I'll be free as a bird. I'll want to do a running jump but contain myself, grabbing my glasses I'll very carefully edge down the staircase arriving at a sliding door. I effortlessly slide it open which is magnificent for me because nothing I do now is ever effortless. I breeze through the opening and shout "surprise" followed by "it's me, Mam and Dad." I'm not sure how they will react but maybe they will doubt who I am and I'll have to prove my identity especially using my spectacles. Eventually they will understand and maybe I'll have to stop one of them falling over after they feel faint. Oh how exhilarating to imagine their stunned reactions as their son is free from his physical prison!

I urge them to keep it a secret for the time being until I surprise my sisters with the news. If it was Sunday they'd both be home so borrowing my mother's trainers (hopefully a near fit) I head outside. I start to run feeling the breeze tug at my hair and face, I make my way to Sian's house. Knocking the door I'm greeted by her and again she probably at first won't recognize me so I'll have to prove myself. I imagine she would phone my parents and they would let her know it's really Ian. She and Mathew will be so excited and I really look forward to that time. Next I'll quietly see my twin nieces, being careful not to startle them because they have never seen me walk before. After they get used to me I'll pick them up and hold them close, giving them the kisses which I ache to do now.

After an emotional visit with Sian and Mathew, where hopefully I'll be allowed to borrow my brother-in-law's spare clothes, I'll head out. This time I'll run to my sister Emma's house where presumably I'll go through the same verification process as before. The reactions will be brilliant to behold and I look forward to my other niece and my nephew's shocked amazement. Nia will proclaim that I now have my working legs and may give me a big hug. I'm really not sure what Iwan will do but they both would probably want me to play games with them and generally keep me busy. Also I am not very sure how my brother-in-law Ceri will react but I'm sure he will be extremely surprised. I'll probably have a long conversation with them, Emma would possibly ring my mother to check that this was me after all and not a dream.

I would then traipse home physically and emotionally drained ready to eat some actual normal food. I would probably have a veritable feast of bread, meat, vegetables and fruits all washed down with water and maybe some wine. I would savour every mouthful exploring all the textures and nuances of these varied morsels. Yummy. The rest of the day would probably go by in a blur of letting my friends and the Church know and putting up status messages on social media. Then delightfully I would go straight to bed because I can cough again without needing a suction machine! I would tentatively drop off without a ventilator whirring away in the corner a little worried that this was all a dream. Thankfully I would wake up and my new life would continue.

Throughout the following days I'd really want to get some new clothes and I'm hoping my father would take me to Cardiff. I haven't been in a car for many years save for my van which is different to a family saloon. It'll be very novel travelling in a car freely able to move without a wheelchair encumbering me. In my current condition I have trouble keeping my head up and moving it in any direction is impossible. Being healed would really free me up and I'd probably have a difficult time staying still! If the sun were low on the journey to the city I could use my hand to shield my eyes which would be a sheer luxury in my present state. After parking the car we'd begin our walk towards the city centre high street taking in all the sights and sounds of the hustle bustle.

I would first buy some comfortable shoes and some formal shoes to replace my mother's purple trainers. It'll be fun seeing what walking feels like in a variety of different shoe styles. After getting the footwear sorted out it'll be time to find some clothes shops especially places with suits. Since I have a pocket watch collection, I really would like a three piece suit with a waistcoat so I can wear my watches on special occasions. I may even try finding a vintage suit to better look the part. I'd obviously need some more casual clothing because you can't wear suits for every occasion. I wouldn't want to go crazy buying clothes - I just want enough to cover my daily needs. Wearing properly fitting clothes is just a dream now but in this daydream anything is possible.

Another novelty would be washing and cleaning myself in total privacy which is extremely rare if not non existent in my present reality. Having a shower all to myself and cleaning up without a carer present would help me feel empowered. Drying myself afterwards would also be entirely novel because I can gauge the exact pressure needed so as not to hurt my body. You may wonder how my tracheotomy tube might endure a shower but hopefully it would be removed by then. The last time I had a short period without a tracheotomy tube the actual hole healed over remarkably quickly. Hopefully this would happen again although it would need covering temporarily with a suitable dressing while it heals.

That leads me to the moment I will tell my respiratory nurses and consultant. They will be blown away in shock and hopefully give me advice on what to do regarding my now removed tracheotomy tube. I can imagine them wanting to contact the media but I really wouldn't want major attention because I get shy. I'd have to arrange to give my ventilators back and return any unused supplies back to their department. To other departments I would return my wheelchair, hoists, hospital bed, lift and all the miscellaneous things that accumulate living the DMD life. My bedroom would be so bare which would take some getting used to, no doubt. I'd even have to buy a new bed and mattress eventually but temporarily I would use the spare room to sleep in.

Over the weeks and months to come I'd stop my benefit payments because I must inform the relevant department of a change in circumstances. That would be quite some conversation where I'd have to explain this miraculous healing. Hopefully they would believe me and allow me to cut the strings to the benefit system. No more jumping through bureaucratic hoops to get financial help will definitely be liberating. I'd then start looking for a job which may prove difficult with my lack of qualifications but I'd work almost anywhere to start with. I'm hoping it'll be somewhere that will fully use my art abilities like a jewellery shop for instance. It'll daunting stepping out into the world of work for the first time because it's a tough place out there. Hopefully I'll adjust to the demands with my family and Church friends supporting me along with faith in God.

There'll be many numerous things and new experiences awaiting me out there but describing them all would require a big book. I definitely want to physically go to Church services instead of using technology every week, although I'm grateful for what I have been given now. I may go travelling depending on my financial situation and learning to drive is absolutely something I want to do. Freedom will be truly magnificent and awesome! There maybe alternative ways I'll be healed and it may involve my death first but eventually my dream will come true. Never stop dreaming is my advice to you dear reader.

# *Acknowledgments*

I'd like to thank all my family for being such good sports all through my writing adventure. Thanks to my Mother for all the care and Pepsi Max she gave me along the way. Recently I lost my grandmother, she will be greatly missed. I'd like to give special thanks to my dear friend Pauline Brace, whose support and early encouragement helped me write this book. Thank you for reading every chapter as I wrote them. Thanks to my current doctors for helping me stay alive so far. All thanks to my God for giving me the gifts and knowledge to write this book and the ability to enjoy the process. Lastly thanks go to you the reader.

I no longer celebrate xmas, Easter or birthdays, so please forgive the references I made to these events as they were part of my life back then.

Lightning Source UK Ltd.
Milton Keynes UK
UKHW041301250820
368797UK00002BA/780

9 781907 652332